Close Enough
Nutrition

Close Enough Nutrition

Eat Nutritiously Using the Dietary Guidelines for Americans for About $5 a Day

Judy Webb Brewster

authorHOUSE®

AuthorHouse™ LLC
1663 Liberty Drive
Bloomington, IN 47403
www.authorhouse.com
Phone: 1-800-839-8640

Published by AuthorHouse   07/19/2013

ISBN: 978-1-4817-7888-6 (sc)
ISBN: 978-1-4817-7889-3 (e)

Library of Congress Control Number: 2013913039

This book is not intended as a substitute for the advice and care of your physician or other health care provider, and you should not undertake any changes in diet without first consulting them. The material in this book is provided for information only and contains the opinions and ideas of the author.

The author expressly disclaims all responsibility for any liability loss, or risk, personal or otherwise, or adverse effects that may result from or is incurred as a consequence, arising directly or indirectly, from the use of application or the information from any of the contents contained in this book.

Any people depicted in stock imagery provided by Thinkstock are models, and such images are being used for illustrative purposes only.
Certain stock imagery © Thinkstock.

This book is printed on acid-free paper.

Because of the dynamic nature of the Internet, any web addresses or links contained in this book may have changed since publication and may no longer be valid. The views expressed in this work are solely those of the author and do not necessarily reflect the views of the publisher, and the publisher hereby disclaims any responsibility for them.

CONTENTS

Acknowledgments

To my wonderful family: husband, daughter, son, son-in-law, both grandsons, both brothers, their wives and families. My parents, grandparents, aunts and uncles and cousins. They all helped shape my personality and my wonderful, amazing outlook on life in general.

I want to especially thank my daughter and son for their love and support through the years. They have always been there for me and have brought me so much pride and joy. I wouldn't have made it without them.

Chapter 1

Ignorance is Not Bliss

If you eat, say, 5,000 calories a day, would you like to know that at least 3,000 of those calories met the nutritional guidelines of the Dietary Guidelines for Americans (DGA) that are paid for by your hard-earned taxes? You can.

I've studied the 2005 and the 2010 Dietary Guidelines for Americans over the last few years. Both are online. I printed them out and then made lists, lots of lists. Those Guidelines were not an easy read for the average Judy.

But, I think I've come close enough to understanding what I need to do in order to meet their recommendations and eat better than I ever have (more like my mother always wanted me too) without giving up all my comfort foods. The Dietary Guidelines are based on a lot of scientific evidence. They used the word, preponderance, which I had to look up, and then I decided on the words, a lot, instead.

The information in my book, Close Enough Nutrition, is based on what I thought was the easiest way to implement their recommendations within my ability to comprehend what I read. So, if I were you, I'd definitely go online and study them yourself at www. dietaryguidelines.gov.

Close Enough Nutrition is not about taking away all white food. It's not about eating mostly protein. It's not about a kitchen stocked with red pepper to crush, black pepper to crack, or tarragon leaves. And it is definitely not about peeling a pound of yuca for a recipe. This book doesn't have recipes. My spice rack has only salt and pepper in it and there's been some controversy about the salt.

What this book does have is more than just saying you need two to three cups of this and three ounces of that to meet your goal. I mean, how do I figure out how to have seventeen grams of oil? I need something more concrete than that. There are no forbidden foods or restrictions in this book. It's not about free days or strict ratios and definitely not a three phase plan of eat this, then eat that and last of all—eat this and that.

This book contains information about what I've collected and was able to put to use on a Daily Nutrition Spreadsheet (DNS) I designed. It has different calorie level scenarios from 1,000 to 3,000 calories in 500 calorie increments. Over the last ten years the spreadsheet went through several revisions before I settled on the current one. Yes, go ahead and look for it. They are in the back of the book (DNS 1 through 5). Even if you are one of those people who read things from front to back, go ahead and look. I think it will help you understand the first chapters better when you know how the information will be applied.

I realized that the best and easiest way to put some more of my hard-earned tax dollars to work was to use the Nutrition Facts label as a reference tool. Later on I decided to combine my food for the day to come as close as I could to reach the 2005 Dietary Guidelines I had found online in 2006. As time passed, and the 2010 Dietary Guidelines came out in 2011, I studied it. Information on fresh food was a little tougher, but doable.

However, the Nutrition Facts (NF) label has a size problem. The government is okay with putting just some of the required information on the can or package if it is too small for everything. I had a different problem with it. It showed only the 2,000 and sometimes the 2,500 calorie levels. My math skills have never been good even though I'll never be able to forget the times tables I learned in grade school. Fractions were never my strong point, but I persevered with a calculator in my hand.

So ten years ago, when all I had to use was the Nutrition Facts label, I purchased a few 28X22 white poster boards to make a chart to track the food I ate. I was surprised when the chart filled up the whole poster. And it was a complicated chart, for me at least. Across the top I put the NF label's list of items like calories, cholesterol, sodium, and protein in a separate column for each one. I included the most referenced vitamins and minerals which were vitamin A and C, plus calcium and iron. Later I added other columns for myself to use for things that I wanted to track.

Down the first column at the left, I listed the different categories from the old USDA Pyramid from the 1990s. I named the first row bread, cereal, and rice. The second row was fruits, the third vegetables. Then I added the milk and cheese row, then the meat, eggs, beans, and nuts row. At the top of the Pyramid were the fats, oils, and sweets for my final row. I left some space between each of these rows to add the foods I regularly ate and wanted to find out about.

When I found the 2005 Dietary Guidelines for Americans I saw that it had different names for the food groups than the 1990s Pyramid. So I made another using those names which were grains, vegetables, fruits, dairy, protein, and oils. On another poster I wrote down information from the DGA I didn't understand in hopes I would eventually figure it out. These included Energy Producing Nutrients and Acceptable Macronutrient Distribution Ranges. Like I said before, the DGA is a hard read for the average Judy. That's why my book is so short.

In the end, I wanted the DNS to provide the approximate daily nutritional energy suggested by the DGA. I wanted to eat as healthy as possible. I don't want to shorten my life or lower the quality of it by not choosing what I eat with more care. That's my motivation.

Again, in my kitchen, you won't find fresh chives that need snipped or baby arugula, or capers, and nothing extra-virgin will ever be in there. Partly it's because I'm not sure how to cook with them. That's why on my kitchen shelves I have things like canned squash, spinach, white and sweet potatoes, carrots, navy beans, salmon, tuna, chicken, and my personal favorite, Mandarin oranges—it's a smorgasbord. They're easier to use with my Daily Nutrition Spreadsheet too.

Although I've heard that ignorance is bliss, I think that the Dietary Guidelines for Americans has given me the power and knowledge to understand how to take the information from the Nutrition Facts label to help me implement my personal food goals, and eventually to make healthier choices each day.

So I highly recommend that you read both the 2005 and the 2010 Dietary Guidelines for Americans in addition to this book or any other book, magazine or internet literature. I hope you will find your own understanding of what the DGAs are trying to tell you about nutrition and how what you eat can affect your health and well being.

So if you want to get off the diet-go-round of low carbohydrates, or low fat, or pills that have inconvenient side effects, and start riding the Rainbow Colored Carousel of the food Pyramid, I urge you to start now. I want all to get the most value out of their life by eating as nutritionally as possible.

And always, always, consult with your physician or other appropriate health care provider to get their okay before trying any new eating plan or even new supplements. This book is only intended to let you know what I discovered for myself about how I wanted to eat and hope it might be helpful to those who read it. Life is a learning curve and I never know whether I'm going up the curve or down it. Other times it seems like there is more than one curve I've been traveling on in this life.

Although I want to eat as healthy as possible, I'm not one to do anything associated with deprivation. And it seems like restricting one's choices of what to eat comes with the word, diet. So this book is called Close Enough Nutrition. That's the best this average Judy can do and still feel I have some freedom to choose what I eat, how I live, and to enjoy what I can within the choices this world gives us.

Chapter 2

What I Discovered

I discovered that there are three items in the Dietary Guidelines for Americans and on the Nutrition Facts label that do not contribute to calories. They are cholesterol, sodium, and potassium. Their milligrams per day for the average healthy adult, 19 plus years old, has limits set by the DGA.

The limit for cholesterol is less than 300 milligrams (mg) daily. When I first heard about this limit a few years ago, the talk was about how one egg a day would reach your limit because it had 300 mg in it. You wouldn't be able to eat anything else that day that contained cholesterol if you wanted to eat healthy.

However, today if you look at the NF label on some egg cartons, you can find a cholesterol level of 215 mg or less. I even found eggs that had 180 mg of cholesterol, contained 100 mg of Omega-3, and its mother was fed vegetarian feed that contained no animal fat, animal by-products, preservatives, or antibiotics. She lived cage free too.

The limit for sodium is less than 2,400 mg daily on the Nutrition Facts label which is about one teaspoon of salt. Again, this is for healthy adults 19 plus years old. The 2010 DGA covers healthy eating information for specific populations too and the recommendations are different for each of them on practically everything. The specific populations are children and adolescents, older adults who are 50 to 70 years old, and those who are 71 plus years old. There are recommendations for women who are capable of becoming pregnant, who are pregnant, and those who are breastfeeding.

There's even information for adults at high risk of chronic disease. And this time the 2010 DGA has included information for vegetarians and vegans too. So for those in specific populations, I think you would want to study the DGA for yourself to understand how to meet your daily recommended nutritional needs.

The limit for potassium is 3,500 mg daily based on the Nutrition Facts label which is the amount I use on my DNS. I had a hard time reaching those limits within the calories I ate to maintain my weight. Then I read in the 2010 DGA that it recommended 4,700 mg. The Appendix 12 in the 2010 DGA has a list of foods that shows the high to low amounts of potassium in them. To reach the 4,700 mg level in a day, using the food with the most potassium in it, I would need to eat just over six small baked potatoes with flesh and skin (each with 738 mg of potassium). In the appendix, the potato averaged 128 calories each which would total 768 calories. I eat between 1,200 and 1,500 calories a day due to my small stature. So that meant half of my food for that day would be potatoes. Yuk.

Other potassium foods, listed in descending order were canned prune and carrot juice, tomato paste, and cooked beet greens, on down to cooked kidney beans at 358 mg of potassium. The orange juice in my refrigerator has 450 mg of potassium in an eight fluid ounce serving. That's just over 10 cups I'd need, with a calorie count of 1,100. Bananas are a good source of potassium. I would need to eat eleven medium bananas at 422 mg which would be 1,155 calories. So I will stick with the NF label of 3,500 mg daily as my reference and do the best I can to get close enough.

———◦◦◦◦———

I discovered there are four energy producing nutrients which are fat, carbohydrates, fiber, and protein. I always thought energy came from sugar and it made little kids hyper when they ate too much. It turns out a carbohydrate does contain sugar, plus starch.

Fats have a bad name. It also has many different names that show up on the Nutrition Facts label. It took a lot of time to track all of them for each food I ate during the day. The recommended fat amount is less than 65 gm at the 2,000 calorie level. On the NF label there is the top section called total fat that shows the grams and the Daily Value percentage. Underneath that is four more sections which shows the amount for saturated fat, trans fat, polyunsaturated fat, and monounsaturated fat. Each one has its own level of grams and percentages.

I struggled with trying to make sense out of how to apply the fat information to my Daily Nutrition Spreadsheet. It became too much for this average Judy. So I have used just the total fat grams for it. If the other fats are something you want to, or need to track, you may enjoy reading the Dietary Guidelines for that information. I found it fascinating how the different fats work in the body. You might too.

Carbohydrates are listed on the NF label as a top section with two indented sections below it which are dietary fiber and sugars that are contained in the carbohydrate. The amount on the NF label is less than 300 grams a day.

Dietary fiber is the non-digestible part of the carbohydrates. I discovered that it takes more than the usual six to eight cups of water a day to give food waste a smooth ride through the intestines. I thought moisture should be enough. I thought wrong. After making sure that I got very close to the recommended amount of fiber in my meals each day, I understood regularity much better.

Non-digestible fiber means it can't be digested as it passes through our digestive tract. The enzymes in there can only dissolve the other parts of the food. The non-digestible fiber is what really keeps things moving along. Popcorn, oatmeal, whole wheat, rice, vegetables, and whole fruits are some of the fiber-rich foods you can consume to reach the recommended level of 25 grams for the average healthy adult on a 2,000 calorie level. Navy beans topped the list at 9.5 grams with the most fiber but that legume is almost non-existent on restaurant menus. As for fruits, a small raw pear has one whole gram more of fiber than the proverbial apple a day.

I happily discovered that the preferred energy source for the brain is sugar and starches. And the body's response is the same whether they are naturally present or added to the food. However, sugar has gotten a bad name too. When I grew up we had three meals a day, cooked at home by my mother, we drank a glass of milk at every meal, and dessert was mostly for birthdays and holidays. We had a garden too.

My children had what we called the Goody Drawer. I kept it supplied with Ding Dongs, Ho Ho's, Twinkies, and other packaged treats. On Sundays we baked chocolate chip cookies or chocolate cake to go with our home-made chocolate ice cream using cream from a cow, not the store-bought kind. For many years we also had three home-cooked meals a day which were later supplemented by what could be cooked in the microwave. We also had a garden.

These days I have a Goody Shelf in my kitchen cabinets for my variety of packaged cookies and candy. My Goody Shelf in the refrigerator's freezer holds a one-half gallon container of Blue Bell's Pecan Pralines 'n Cream at 190 calories per one-half cup. Its first two ingredients in the list are milk and cream. Oh yeah.

My daughter has a Goody Drawer in her refrigerator. Whenever I kept my two grandsons when my daughter and son-in-law were on a business trip, I would feed them their after school snacks from it. Inside were fresh broccoli and cauliflower to dip in yogurt. She is not adopted.

If you think, or your physician or health care provider says, you need to watch your sugar intake, here is one of the ways you can by using the Nutrition Facts label. The grams on the label help you keep track of it. I think it would help if you at least read that section of the DGA for yourself too.

To help you in your decisions when adding sugar to your food, it takes one teaspoon of sugar to equal 4 grams. And one teaspoon equals 15 calories.

So a little sugar may be good for the brain, but some prepared foods add sugar to make the taste more palatable. We now seem to be overdoing a good thing. The NF label has just the amount of total sugar grams listed on it. It doesn't show the added sugars as different from the naturally occurring sugars, it's just the total of any sugars. One should study the ingredients of the food on the label very carefully. They are supposed to be listed in descending order first by the ingredient with the most weight on down to the least amount of weight which is listed last and this information may influence what food you choose.

Protein makes me think of chickens, turkeys, pigs, and cows. However, it also comes from plant foods like beans and 'eat your peas' plus soy products, seeds, and nuts. I'm using the NF label information for protein which is 50 grams on the 2,000 calorie level for average healthy adults.

The information on protein is another reason I decided to use just the NF label for my spreadsheet. The 2010 Dietary Guidelines for Americans has the recommended amounts for protein as five one-half ounce-equivalents on the 2,000 calorie level. Then it lists a sub-group of protein foods and their ounces that you can use to reach your nutritional needs over a week's time. I had a brain freeze about then and decided to just KISS it. Keep It Simple and Sensible.

The last thing I discovered was the Acceptable Macronutrient Distribution Ranges, aka the AMDRs. These listed the range of percentages of the total calories for three groups based on a 2,000 calorie level. Said another way, it is the recommended percent per day on a 2,000 calorie level for fat, carbohydrates, and protein.

Based on the 2005 Dietary Guidelines for Americans they are:

> 20 to 35% of Fat
> 45 to 65% of Carbohydrates
> 10 to 35% of Protein

Based on the 2010 Dietary Guidelines for Americans for Adults (19 years up) they are:

> 20 to 35% of Fat
> 45 to 65% of Carbohydrates
> 10 to 35% of Protein

The only difference between the two examples above is the specification in the 2010 DGA where it defines the parameters for an adult. It also listed the percentages for young children (1-3 years) and older children and adolescents (4-18 years). I avoid doing percentages as much as possible, even with a calculator, so I used grams and milligrams instead. And for those who may want to know, or don't know and won't ask, one gram equals 1,000 milligrams.

Then I read about my two biggest discoveries. The first one was in a section in the 2010 DGA, on page 15 in Chapter Two. The Institute of Medicine (IOM) is the agency that established the ranges for the AMDRs. It stated that, "The total number of calories consumed is the essential dietary factor relevant to body weight."

It also pointed out that, "Strong evidence shows that there is no optimal proportion of macronutrients that can facilitate weight loss or assist with maintaining weight loss. Although diets with a wide range of macronutrient proportions have been documented to promote weight loss and prevent weight regain after loss, evidence shows that the critical issue is not the relative proportion of macronutrients in the diet, but whether or not the eating pattern is reduced in calories and the individual is able to maintain a reduced-calorie intake over time."

The second one was in the 2005 Dietary Guidelines for Americans on page VII, which stated, "However, even following just some of the recommendations can have health benefits." That, to me, is their version of the KISS method. Keep It Simple and Sensible. That's what I wanted to convey with my book, Close Enough Nutrition.

Chapter 3

Nutrients, Vitamins, and Minerals

From what I gathered as an average Judy from the 2005 and 2010 Dietary Guidelines for Americans, food nutrients are measured in grams, milligrams, and ounces. They are the ones that have the calories. The total calories of these nutrients, per serving, are listed on the Nutrition Facts label. Vitamins and minerals are measured in international units, milligrams, and micrograms. The NF label doesn't list them that way. It has each one listed as a Daily Value percentage based on a 2,000 calorie level. So when the amount for them reaches the 100% mark, you have fulfilled the recommended level for that day.

So if the food you're eating has a NF label that lists vitamin A as 25% per serving, then somewhere in your daily 2,000 calorie food intake you need 75% more vitamin A to meet the recommended level. If your daily food intake is 1,500 calories, then 75% of that 100% is all you need and so on. For my Daily Nutrition Spreadsheet I had a hard time deciding how to represent the vitamins and minerals to reflect each of the different calorie levels. I do so dislike doing fractions.

Also, because no matter what calorie level you find you want to come close enough to, the Nutrition Facts label's information will always be based on that 100%. That becomes a ridiculous amount of fractions to remember to change for each item you eat every day. So on the DNS I have in this book, you will see that I have put under the columns for them, a box with an explanation. It says, "Percent totals at the top of these columns are for the 100% on the NF label needed at 2,000 calories." That's the best this average Judy can do. You can lay out your spreadsheet however it works best for you.

On my spreadsheet I eventually added one more row at the very top and named it Total Daily Nutrition. It has the totals for all of the columns. I put it up there instead of at the bottom because of the ease to see the second and third rows below it. The second row has the numbers you want to achieve for the nutrients and the third row has the name of the nutrient. This is the kind of adjustments you can do to your spreadsheet or tracking system to make it personalized for your needs.

The only vitamins and minerals required to be on the NF label are vitamin A, vitamin C, calcium, and iron and these are the ones I have on my Daily Nutrition Spreadsheets to be tracked plus vitamin D. If you don't want to use the Daily Value percentage, then you will want to note that vitamin A is measured in International Units (IUs). Vitamin C, calcium, and iron are measured in milligrams (mg). For the average healthy adult (19 years and older) based on the 2,000 calorie level, vitamin A is 5,000 IU, vitamin C is 60 mg, calcium is 1,000 mg, and iron is 18 mg. Again, the specific populations listed in the 2010 Dietary Guidelines for Americans will have some different recommendation levels.

There is something else you need to be aware of on the NF label's information. There are several foods that have very few of the nutrients that are required to be on the NF label. There is usually a disclaimer in small letters somewhere that uses the words, not a significant source of, and then lists the nutrients.

With all of this in mind, I wanted to list some nutrients, vitamins, and minerals with some information about each of them from the DGA that I think is important, interesting, and easy to understand. I think you can look at this information to help you decide what foods to eat during your day and with the Daily Nutrition Spreadsheet, you can choose the calorie level you want to use.

Let's say that you are not interested in changing the amount of daily calories you have been eating. You are not wanting to diet by reducing what you usually eat in a day. Your objective is trying to choose what you eat so that it is nutritious. Perhaps you want to track your sodium, check your fiber intake, or manage your cholesterol better. Or do you just want to know, like me, an easier way to eat nutritiously most of the time to get close enough to healthy eating. Of course, you can use the Dietary Nutrition Spreadsheet to count your calories to increase or decrease them too, but that option is up to you.

To illustrate the Nutrition Facts label for a bowl of Apple Cinnamon Cheerios, I thought I'd use the 2,000 calorie level example in the format below. Keep in mind that potassium is not required to be on the label whether it is included in the food or not. Now that Vitamin D has started becoming more important, some NF labels have started listing it.

There are labels on some canned and packaged foods that now want you to know they contain or have added Calcium, Vitamin D, Omega-3, and on top of all of that, please notice that they are fat-free too. Never mind that some of them have always been fat-free in the past.

Cheerios NF label		Nutrition Facts label	
Serving size	3/4 cup	Serving size	3/4 cup
Calories per serving	120	Calorie level	2,000

Total fat	1.5 g	Less than	65 g
Trans fat	0g		
Cholesterol	0g	Less than	300g
Sodium	115 mg	Less than	2,400g
Carbohydrate	24g	Less than	300g
Dietary fiber	2g		25g
Sugars	10g		
Protein	2g		50g
Potassium	65 mg		3,500g
Vitamin A	10%	of 5,000 IU	
Vitamin C	10%	of 60 mg	
Calcium	10%	of 1,000 mg	
Iron	25%	of 18 mg	

It's hard to know where to draw the line on the multitude of information on the Nutrition Facts label. On this particular label I couldn't see the value in some of it, since for my purposes, this list was close enough. If you want the extra information for yourself, you can change the DNS format or use another format you design as a guideline.

The Cheerios is just one item in a full day's nutritional food that needs to be eaten. It doesn't even have milk on it yet. I'm going to list what I ate that day in the awful format below that pushed me to realize I needed to figure out how to use a spreadsheet to ease the pain of it all. I ate about 1,250 calories that day. I adjusted the figures from the 2,000 calorie level so I'd know approximately how I matched up with the Dietary Guidelines for Americans at the 1,200 calorie level.

Besides the Cheerios for breakfast, I added one cup of fat-free milk with vitamins A and D, and one sliced medium banana, with one tablespoon of sugar spread over the top of it all. For lunch it was two tablespoons of peanut butter on two slices of whole wheat bread and one tablespoon of seedless strawberry jam. For a snack, I had a medium apple, a slice of cheese, and five ounces of V8 tomato juice.

My evening meal consisted of one slice of whole wheat bread, two ounces of solid white Albacore tuna in water, one hard-boiled egg, and one tablespoon of light salad dressing. I would be close enough to doing my body right that day after adding a cup of fat-free milk with Vitamins A and D, plus one-half cup each of carrots, green beans, and mandarin oranges.

Here comes the best part of the 2005 Dietary Guidelines for Americans for me because I get to enjoy my comfort foods. It's called the Discretionary Calorie Allowance. I looked up discretionary and found that it means I have the power to use my own judgment on what to eat for these calories. So I could decide between three-fourths cup of ice cream at 240 calories or three double stuffed cookies at 210 calories. I do have to say, the DGA had their own choices of what calories I could choose from, but what can I say, they didn't interest me in the least.

I added everything up and compared the results to the DGA at my targeted 1200 calorie level. The following is what it looked like before I came up with the Dietary Nutrition Spreadsheet.

> 34 total fat grams of the allowed 39 gm.
> 284 mg of cholesterol of the less than 300 mg.
> 2025 mg of sodium of the less than 2,400 mg.
> 179 gm of carbohydrates of the allowed 180 gm.
> 18.5 mg of dietary fiber of the needed 15.5 mg.
> 2025 mg of potassium of the needed 3,500 mg.
> 69.5 gm of protein for the allowed 30 gm.
> 113 gm of sugar.
> 265% of vitamin A of the 100% at 2,000 calories.
> 133% of vitamin C of the 100% at 2,000 calories.
> 129% of calcium of the 100% at 2,000 calories.
> 58% of iron of the 100% at 2,000 calories.

This is hard work. It's time consuming when I'd rather be doing other things. However it does come pretty close to the DGA except possibly for the sugar. I have worked on the sugar part since because I became aware of the problem during my study of how I could eat more nutritionally. I knew I ate more sugar than I should but I didn't know it was this gross. Once again, I've discovered ignorance is not bliss. Knowledge is power. Motivation to do better can mean a healthier me.

———⊷⊶⊷———

I eat a lot of the same foods. But the choice of just deciding which can of green beans to purchase can give me a headache. Turns out it's a legume which is a flowering plant with pods that split open. I thought that was just pea pods that were split open to get the peas. And it was green beans that we snapped the ends off before breaking them into three pieces before cooking. It turns out that on the can, they call it cut green beans because from the picture it is obvious something sharp was used to slice it. Now, consider what you have to decide among with just these three brands, Libby's, Green Giant, and Del Monte.

Libby's has what I call a regular can of green beans. Its ingredient list says it contains cut green beans, water, and salt. That's it. The picture on the front shows cut green beans too. Libby's also has the choice of a can of cut green beans that says on the front it doesn't have salt or sugar added. Listed just above its ingredient list of green beans and water are the words, not a sodium free food. So I look at the Nutrition Facts label for sodium and sure enough, 15 mg is listed. The sodium on the other can without this claim has 380 mg listed. So there must be a natural amount of sodium in green beans.

Then I wondered about the sugar. Do green beans have a natural amount of sugar in them? Apparently it's possible since I found it on all six cans I looked at. Each one listed two grams of sugar except one which listed one gram. Libby's was the only one to state that it did not add any sugar to their green beans. Could that be a selling ploy to get our attention if we are watching our sugar intake? I don't know for sure since I'm just the average Judy trying to make a nutritious choice for the food I plan to eat.

Green Giant has their regular can of cut green beans showing the whole bean on the front with a little round inset showing three cut green beans. Its ingredients also list green beans, water, and salt. Its sodium is listed at 400 mg and its serving size is the same as the others, one-half cup. Green Giant also has a can choice that has 50% less sodium than their regular beans. The ingredients list green beans, water, and salt. The sodium is listed at 200 mg.

And then there's Del Monte. They have Blue Lake cut green beans. I don't know what Blue Lake means, I did not look it up, and I only know they were my father's favorite. Its ingredients were green beans, water, and salt. Del Monte's also had a can choice that said it had no salt added. It listed 10 gm of sodium. And, like Libby's, it stated that it was not a sodium-free food.

The good thing about all of this is if you want to or have to watch your sodium intake, you can easily make a decision. All the cans had on their Nutritional Facts label the same amount of 20 calories per serving, and zero fat and cholesterol. After that there were some differences.

I have one more example of how difficult it can be to check the nutrition of the foods you are eating in a day to try and meet the Dietary Guidelines. Take my bitter butter battles. Please.

Let's say I want some butter to spread on my morning toast. Or maybe I want margarine. Sounds simple enough, but a trip to the store had me wishing for some of my in-laws cow cream so I could use the Dazey butter churn from my childhood to make it into just plain butter. At the store I find that one brand asks me to choose between fat free or sweet cream and calcium, a light or a Mediterranean blend. Not even their original comes in one choice. Do I want it in a stick, bowl, or a squeeze bottle which by the way, just happens to come in a new, larger size.

Choosing my breakfast butter has turned into a gargantuan task that is mind-boggling because of the assortment of this one item on the grocery shelf. The brightly colored labels swear at me that there's no trans fat, or its cholesterol free, and now I can have it with 500 mg of Omega-3, plus I could have it fortified with calcium and vitamin D too. Oh, and did I want it salt-free?

Did I give up? No. At least they had concrete information that I could use to make a decent choice and put it on my Daily Nutrition Spreadsheet. All of these choices were better than the information that the Dietary Guidelines gave for a 2,000 calorie level. Their list was two cups of fruit, two and a half cups of vegetables, six ounces of grain, five and a half ounces of protein, three cups of dairy, and twenty-seven grams of oil/fats. So I will happily spend my time looking at the information on the Nutrition Facts labels at the grocery store to decide what foods I'll let pass my lips on its way to become energy for my body.

CHAPTER 4

TIMING IS EVERYTHING

How often should we eat during the day? So many choices and so little time is usually the key to how many of us make that decision. The one most everyone agrees on is that we should eat breakfast after we wake up. That makes sense to me because it's been several hours since you last ate and your body needs some nutrients to use for its energy in order to run at an optimum level for you. I think your lifestyle, your culture, your home life as a child can all enter into our choices of when to eat and then, should you always eat at the table? Some people do and some eat in the car (think fast food) or in their favorite chair in front of the TV.

Sometimes we have no choice at school, at work, or at home because the circumstances require a schedule of some sort. I prefer flexibility rather than making a precise schedule that someone else has designed which, to me, defeats the whole idea of enjoying the food you eat. Then there are those who think you shouldn't eat after five or six or whenever in the evening.

How about six times a day? You could start with breakfast at 7:00 a.m. and then a morning snack at 9:30 a.m. After lunch at noon you could have a snack at 2:30 p.m. followed by dinner at 6 p.m. That leaves you a snack before bedtime at 8:00 p.m. Some people need a schedule due to medical reasons and others because knowing when they will eat is important to them.

I've seen co-workers who snack and eat throughout the day. They call it grazing. It seems to me that their real hunger never gets to show itself as a recognizable need to satisfy. Little babies let you know when they have a recognizable need to satisfy. They know when they are hungry, wet, sick, or just need to burp. And real soon you know it too.

There was a time when parents were encouraged to coax their new little ones into waiting four hours between feeding periods. The next goal was to have them sleep through the night without waking to be fed. Unless there is some medical problem that counteracts waiting four hours between eating something, I think adults might try waiting those four hours. Will they think they will waste away if they don't have something within two hours? Are they having hunger pangs or are they just thirsty. It's so easy to take food with us or get it where ever we are. When we pay at the cash register, do you notice how many areas around it contain snack food? It's there, it's everywhere.

I suggest that you find out what is most suitable for your objectives and lifestyle. If you cook at home or eat out or use prepared food that comes in cans, or frozen packages, or boxes, there is a way to make a schedule that fits you. I think my spreadsheet works well because you can plan ahead of time for each day, or just as eating time comes each day. It's adjustable. After using them for a while, it might come naturally for you to remember what your day needs to round it out to come close enough to eating nutritionally.

How often should we weigh if we're counting calories to increase or decrease our weight to judge how we're doing? Some prefer once every day, morning or night. Some prefer once a week sometimes wearing the same clothes each time or no clothes at all. Some don't want to know and don't own a scale. They just use how their clothes feel on their body.

Weighing every day will let you monitor the fluctuation in your body's processing of food. The daily difference could be one or two pounds or more. It might be water weight gain or loss, or you ate two big meals in a row. It can take about twenty-four hours for food to pass through your system and in some cases forty-eight or more. So unless the scale consistently registers a lower (or higher) number from your original, it's probably just the normal fluctuation you have.

Weighing once a week might have the same hazardous effect. If you want to lose weight and a big meal has just left your body and your water weight is down, you will weigh less and you will feel good about it. Then the next week when you weigh and the situation is the opposite and you weigh more, you will be disappointed. Yet, there's been no actual weight change.

If you decide not to weigh at all, then your clothes will tell you when you have a weight loss or gain. When my last scale quit working, I didn't replace it. When using the scale in the mornings I didn't fluctuate much between two and five pounds, and in spite of myself, I would be disappointed when the scale showed a couple of pounds or more weight gain. So I don't miss the scale at all and stay about the same when weighed at the doctor's office for my annual visit.

So, the choice is up to you. What do you need for motivation? Every day, once a week, or just use your clothes to give you a clue. Try all three to figure it out. Maybe you'll come up with something entirely new, just for you.

———◦◦◦◦———

When should we start an eating plan to be close enough to the Dietary Guidelines? Start on a Monday or on a weekend? Now or tomorrow or when it's convenient? How about after the holidays? How about getting a head start before the holidays?

No matter when you start, you know you want to start. If you don't make it a convenient time for your lifestyle, you won't want to stay started. If you want to sneak up on your eating habits, you can start by reading the labels of everything you are currently eating. I think that when you have a grasp of how you eat now, you'll be better able to see what areas you can keep and what areas you might want to change.

This will also help to find out what calorie range you are in and what amount you want to have to get close enough to the DGA. To me it would be easier to start with just tracking the calories of what you are currently eating for a couple of days, a week or whatever makes you feel comfortable that you have a good daily average calorie count to use.

Then you can start by making a few copies of my Daily Nutrition Spreadsheet to use to list the Nutrition Facts label information on it for each day. You might be able to see a pattern of too much of this or too little of that like I did on the sugar grams.

You can also add columns of your own to track items that you or your doctor thinks is important to your health and well-being. Perhaps add a column for vitamin D or the other fats or even a column for the daily percentage for the Acceptable Macronutrient Distribution Range. At any rate, find your starting place on the road to eating nutritionally using the Dietary Guidelines for Americans and just start.

Chapter 5

Deciphering the 2,000 Calorie Base

Using the Nutrition Facts label for the column headings on my Daily Nutrition Spreadsheet had its tribulations. Decipher is the word I chose to describe what I went through to find a concrete basis for the grams, milligrams, and micrograms used on the Nutrition Facts label. I waded through the 2005 and the 2010 Dietary Guidelines for Americans more than a few times to "make sense of" the information they contained.

Granted, both DGAs are not an easy read for this average Judy, but I even looked at websites (government) at what they had for the Nutrition Facts label to see what I may not have understood. No luck. The DGAs are so careful about the CYA principle, that it wasn't easy to find a common ground for the information for just the average healthy adult (AHA).

Most of the time, the AHA was described as 19 plus years old. But other places the years were from 19 to 50 years old. Oh, and then there's the 50 to 70 and a 70 plus years old category and all of them healthy of course. I struggled on. Again, this is what I came up with for my information. I recommend, strongly, that you also read the DGAs and come to your own conclusions as you plan your way to healthier food choices that come as close as you can to the guidelines.

There's no way I want to adhere exactly to a certain calorie level. The 2010 DGA has a calorie list from 1,000 to 3,200 in increments of 200 calories in their Appendix 7, USDA Food Patterns, on page 79 that you can use for your spreadsheet if you prefer. I used 1,000 to 3,000 in increments of 500 calories in my spreadsheets. That way I had easier fractions for me to make the adjustments for the column headings ;-).

The thing about the DGA list is that they use cups of this, ounce-equivalents of that, and then grams on top of those two for their recommendations. Then they have sub-groups under vegetables, grains, and protein for which they give a weekly amount to reach inside of the main group. Even the above-average Judy would wonder if it's worth all of that work to try to come close enough to eating healthy. The urge to just open the refrigerator door and eat what looks good starts sounding a whole lot easier to do.

With all of that in mind, I decided to start my first column on my Daily Nutritional Spreadsheet as the Serving Size. That is a trickier area than you might imagine on the Nutrition Facts (NF) label. My mind thinks that when I eat a bowl of cereal for breakfast I put in a cup. However, most cereal labels use three-fourths of a cup for their measurement. I don't like to measure anything that closely but in deference to my wish to eat healthy within my target calorie range, I marked my bowl at that level rather than take out a three-fourths measuring cup to pour my cereal in first. Another dirty dish to clean too I might add.

The next column heading, Calories, is much easier to find on the NF label. It's always in the same place and when used in conjunction with the serving size, it's supposed to be accurate.

The next column heading is Fat. I've already complained about the fat category. So I decided for my DNS to use the number by the heading Total Fats on the NF label. If you need or want to track the others, you can add them to your spreadsheet. For the 2,000 calorie level it is recommended to be less than 65 grams. There may be those, with a better math mind than I have, who remember I mentioned that fat is one of the Acceptable Macronutrient Distribution Ranges. They might want to track the percentage in their spreadsheet too. As a reminder, both the 2005 and 2010 DGAs recommended range for fat for any calorie level is 20 to 35%.

Here's one of the easy ones, Cholesterol is part of the fat group. Not only does it not add to the calorie intake, but it is a steady number of less than 300 mg for all calorie levels. However, the less than part can go down if the calories go down from the 2,000 level. The 2005 DGA recommended even less than 200 mg for adults who have elevated LDL, the bad cholesterol. As always, check with your physician or health care provider for their guidance on your health issues.

Sodium, rather than the word salt, is used on the NF label. Salt is sodium chloride and about one teaspoon contains the recommended less than 2,400 mg level of sodium. The less than information is listed not only for sodium and cholesterol on the label, but also for total fat. It's like if you go for less than on any of these items, the DGA will be happy that you did. It reminds me of my motto. "Do your body right and it will do right by you."

For your information, when a RDA (Recommended Dietary Allowance) cannot be determined, the Institute of Medicine (IOM) will set a level for the nutrient. The 2010 DGA goes into detail about this on how IOM sets an Adequate Intake (AI) level for these nutrients. The IOM also has a Tolerable Upper Intake Level (UL). Again, lots of detail about the amount for each age group and please read it if you want to know about your personal needs. It set the UL level at 2,300 mg per day for sodium. However, I'm using the FDA Nutrition Facts label for my DNS and it sets it at less than 2,400 mg.

Carbohydrates are an energy producing nutrient. Like fat they are also in the Acceptable Macronutrient Distribution Range in the DGAs for 45% to 65% of any calorie level. The NF label has it listed as 300 gm (grams) based on the 2,000 calorie level and I will be using grams for my spreadsheet (keeping in mind my fraction problem).

Carbohydrates include sugar (which doesn't have a % Daily Value on the NF label) and starches (not on the NF label at all). It also has fiber which is listed at 25 gm (grams) on the NF label for the 2,000 calorie level.

Speaking of Fiber and its 25 grams for the 2,000 calorie level and that it's part of the carbohydrates. Depending on your digestive needs, you might want to check out the 2010 DGA's Appendix 13 on page 88 that lists the standard portion size of a food along with the dietary fiber in that portion size. I will use the NF label for the gram level on my DNS depending on the calorie level chosen to come close enough to the Dietary Guidelines.

Protein is another one that doesn't have a % Daily Value on the NF label. Protein does have 50 grams listed for the 2,000 calorie level on the NF label which is what I use on my DNS sheets for the average healthy adult.

Although not required on the NF label, I put Potassium in one of my columns because I haven't been able to reach the recommended amount. I may never reach it consistently, but I want to come as close as possible.

And here is where choosing between the foods I want to eat, versus the food I need to eat that day, can become a necessary evil unless I can incorporate it into my designated calorie level. Take potato chips versus baked potatoes. The chips I eat have 350 mg potassium in a one ounce serving of about 15 chips with 160 calories. One small baked potato with flesh and skin has 738 mg of potassium with 128 calories.

It looks like the baked potato wins hands down. But not if for my fruit that day I have a half-cup of apricots (756 gm) as a snack and for breakfast a banana (422 gm) and a cup of milk (382 gm) on my Cheerios (160 mg) along with a cup of my orange juice (450 gm). That's a total of 2,170 grams of potassium toward the NF label of 3,500 grams.

I have a good start to get close enough to my level of potassium that day to enjoy my chips (350 gm) with my chicken (237 gm) and cheese (180 gm) sandwich on whole wheat bread for lunch. Final total even before the evening meal is 2,937 grams of potassium to go toward the target goal of 3,500 grams. How about that? This is the kind of planning you can do in order to do your body right and still enjoy some potato chips.

Sugar is the last column before the vitamins and minerals. I've already said enough about this item. You can track it and use the information for your own purposes as needed.

The DGA didn't go into detail on vitamins except a little about Vitamin D and B12. Remember, choosing nutrients that come primarily from foods gives the body a natural supply of vitamins and minerals and other substances. So if you have any questions on supplements or other additions or subtractions of any kind, please discuss it with you doctor or health care provider.

I also want to remind you to remember to look at another part of the Nutrition Facts label when choosing your food. It's the ingredient list. As much as I try, there is something I add to my coffee that tastes good but the ingredients sound awful. You would think that knowing this would stop me but it doesn't. But I don't berate myself for it either. This average Judy is only human and does the best she can.

The ingredient list is sugar, vegetable oil (partially hydrogenated coconut or palm kernel, hydrogenated soybean), corn syrup solids, and less than 2% of sodium caseinate (a milk derivative) natural and artificial flavors, dipotassium phosphate (moderates coffee acidity), mono and diglycerides (prevents oil separation) salt, sodium aluminosilicate, sucralose. Yummy.

CHAPTER 6

CAPTURING GRAMS AND MILLIGRAMS

The Dietary Guidelines for Americans gives science-based advice on food choices. However, words on paper don't always transfer well into a daily life situation. I couldn't see where the DGA words transferred at all into the grocery store.

Even with what appears to be all of that wonderful, concrete information on the Nutrition Facts label, it left a lot to be desired when trying to put together a cohesive daily food plan. Eating healthy is hard to do. Taking the time to plan to eat healthy is even harder to do in my opinion.

Back when I started all of this, I decided I needed to bring out another one of my 28X22 white poster boards to take a crack at organizing a feasible eating plan. The first try was a mess and so the poster board hit the trash can. However, it did help to foster an idea for my next try at capturing the illusive grams and milligrams.

If you have children and they make the mistake of saying they are bored and have nothing to do, the following information on how to eat nutritiously would keep them busy for a while. It might even become a game to see who can put together the most meals at the different calorie levels chosen by each member of the family.

I started by taking all the labels off the food cans. After they were empty of course, unlike when newlywed couples were given a shivaree (look it up if you don't know what it means) and one of the fun parts was removing the labels on full cans. Then later on I sorted them in like groups used in the DGA. I put each group into a file folder and labeled them Fruits, Vegetables, Grains, Protein, Dairy, and Oils. Oils gave me a problem for a while until I realized they meant Fats. So I put the labels from my cookie and candy packages in there.

I found that if I really wanted to I could use almost all canned food to get my daily nutrients. Since I don't cook, I thought what a great idea. And then I thought of a name for this book. I decided to call it Can Your Diet. But then I realized that it would make too many dull daily meals for the average Judy. So I started saving labels from frozen and packaged foods too.

When I had collected several days' worth of labels, I went back to my poster board. It took two more of these to add this part of my research on how to eat healthy to get close enough to meeting the nutrition needs on the NF label. I added way to many columns in my first layout. Filling out each column for each label took a long time. But then at the end, while admiring my work, I could see why I now needed to put this information into a spreadsheet on my computer. That way I could add or subtract the food information to get a total for the column as I put each food in to see what I needed to adjust, (DNS 6 through 15).

I also found that it worked better if I could decide what I wanted, or was going to have, for my main meal of the day. Then I could build the rest of the day around it. Lots of time was involved at first. Then I could see patterns and started remembering and recognizing what food would work best for my day.

It was easier for me since I eat a lot of the same foods every day and I don't cook. You might look at starting this way too until you start remembering the information. For a lot of us, our breakfast foods are pretty consistent. There are usually three or four kinds of ingredients. There's the cereal, milk, toast, and juice for one. The cereal can be microwavable oatmeal, or cereal with lots of fiber, or cereal for fun, or a favorite like mine—Apple Cinnamon Cheerios.

The toast can be bagels, muffins, specialty bread like sourdough or cinnamon raisin wheat bread. Your choice of dairy might be yogurt or cheese instead of milk on your cereal. Juice could be applesauce or peaches instead of orange or white grape juice (my favorite). This is another way to use my KISS method, keep it simple and sensible.

A main meal for me is usually a sandwich with accouterments. I love that word and it's a rare place that it can be worked into the conversation. It means accessories, trimmings, bits and pieces and last but not least, side dishes. Earlier I had rationalized how eating potato chips can be just as good as a baked potato. I like the crunchy sound effects too. I can add fruit or vegetables to the main meal to round it out. More than likely, I'll also add a cookie or two to make the afternoon go better.

Another main meal for me is a frozen dinner to microwave. These are really easy to lay out in the spreadsheet and add other accouterments to it. A lot of them contain the protein (chicken), vegetables (broccoli or carrots), fruit (as in caramel apple dessert), and even sweet potatoes. Frozen meals usually have around 250 to 350 calories for the whole meal.

I still advise at first, to begin tracking your food to just keep the calorie count. Don't do or eat anything different until you have a good daily average of calories in order to use the Daily Nutrition Spreadsheet nearest that calorie amount. You'll also be able to accumulate many Nutrition Facts labels. Be sure and keep enough of the label to show what the food is too. Not that I had any problem, but wanted to warn you that it can happen.

One other easy way to sneak up on this time consuming effort of tracking what you eat is to add a column or two at a time of information for a while. Say you know that you want to keep track of your cholesterol intake. You know it should be less than 300 milligrams a day. If you add to that the column for fiber, 25 grams, you will have the calories, fiber, and cholesterol information for each day if you are using the 2,000 calorie level spreadsheet.

Habit begins to take over and now you might be curious as to how many carbohydrates and protein you are eating each day. After tracking these too, you will find out which one of any of these items need adjusting, up or down, to come close enough to the Dietary Guidelines for Americans without giving up all of your comfort foods.

By now, I think you would be ready make an effort to add in information for all of the columns you want to track. Some of you will want to fill in as many of the columns as you can for the day before you eat any meal. Some of you will fill it in as the day progresses. Either way, see how you feel at the end of those days where you have tracked your food intake to come close to the DGA. Hopefully, it will be better than you have usually felt since the energy you are feeding your body is right, so your body can then do right by you.

When I look at a box of cereal to purchase and I see something that says it contains 22 grams of whole grain per serving, I think oh good, lots of fiber. But when I look at the fiber content per serving on the NF label, it says three grams. My mind played a trick on me when I didn't put two and two together correctly. My first thought was that I was getting 22 grams of fiber because that's what whole grain means to me. But it really meant 22 grams of whole grain which I guess works down to three grams of fiber per their serving size after processing. I don't really know. This box was one of those one-serving size boxes.

So then I looked at my regular size box of Apple Cinnamon Cheerios which said it had 14 grams of grain per serving and it contained two grams of fiber. Here again, I found I needed to look at the serving size. My regular box had the usual serving size of most cereals at three-fourths cup (30g) and the calories were 120. The serving size on the little box just said 1 box (26g) and 100 calories.

I wondered if the four gram difference in the small serving size box was the reason it was 20 calories less. So then I go to the ingredient list on each box. The small box of Cheerios listed its first ingredient as whole grain oats. Then some corn starch, sugar, salt, phosphate, wheat starch and vitamin E.

The regular size Apple Cinnamon Cheerios box had some extra sugar. The first ingredient was whole grain oats. The next ingredients were sugar, brown sugar, corn meal, corn starch, and corn syrup. After those came a few other things but no more sugar. So of course I look at the Nutrition Facts label for the sugar grams. It was one gram for the regular Cheerios and 10 grams for the Apple Cinnamon Cheerios. My detective skills paid off. If I am watching my sugar intake, I can make a better choice of what food to eat by reading the NF label thoroughly.

Following is the last cereal example of why tracking grams and fiber and sugar can drive you up a wall. It's also why I think everything should just be written down on the Daily Nutrition Spreadsheet with the only goal being to have all the foods that day come as close as possible to the Dietary Guidelines. Never mind how you got there.

Froot Loops are also made with whole grain as the box states and it also states it's a good source of fiber. However, its first ingredient is sugar. This is also a one box serving size with 27 grams and 100 calories. The fiber is three grams like the regular Cheerios which is good. The sugar is 11 grams, only one more gram than the Apple Cinnamon Cheerios that had whole grain oats as its first ingredient. Go figure. Should the Apple Cinnamon Cheerios have had sugar as their first ingredient too? Since I'm tracking only the total grams, then it doesn't matter what I eat as long as I stay within my target nutrition range for the day.

⎯⎯⎯⎯◦◦◦◦⎯⎯⎯⎯

When I look at a jar of peanut butter to purchase and I see on the label something that says seven grams of natural protein, I think well, that sounds good. Turns out, unlike the confusion I had with the box of cereal, the Nutrition Facts label also says seven grams of protein—although the word natural is left out. So to my mind, natural could mean that the two peanuts that have grown up inside their comfy shell are considered a natural food and that's what I'll be eating.

But then I look at the ingredient list. The first words are roasted peanuts. The next word is sugar and at the end of the list is salt. In between the sugar and salt is the type of oil the peanuts were roasted in and another ingredient to prevent separation. Apparently they didn't know about an ingredient to prevent separation yet for peanut butter when I was growing up.

I liked stirring in the oily stuff with a dinner knife before spreading the peanut butter on my white bread since eating whole wheat bread was non-existent back then too. It also took great skill to spread the stiff peanut butter onto the bread without tearing it apart. Today's peanut butter is like spreading canned icing on a cake.

Our school lunches, for twenty-five cents a day, sometimes included hot rolls freshly baked that morning. Our picnic-like lunch tables had big half-gallon cans of peanut butter sitting on them alongside a bottle of white syrup. I added the syrup to a huge mound of peanut butter on my plate and stirred it all up to put on my hot rolls. The rest of the time I put my tasty mixture on regular white bread that was also on the table. Then I ate as much as I could of the food the servers put on my sectioned plastic plate when I went through the lunch line.

There weren't any Nutrition Facts labels back then. There wasn't any concern about obesity in adults, much less children, back then. There wasn't any fast food drive through restaurant chains then either. We can't go back to the good old days. Most of us wouldn't want to anyway. All we can do is gather the best information we can to cope with today's world as it is. The NF labels help us eat as close as we can nutritionally, by using the Dietary Guidelines for Americans scientific-based advice to show us how.

———⬦⬦⬦⬦———

Here's a little bit more about nuts and their grams. It always has been a cholesterol free food with zero grams of trans fat. But now you will also find these words on food labels in what I perceive as an incentive to buy that product over others even though the other product is the same.

Nuts have protein. Protein has fat. Fat has calories. Protein has four calories per gram. Fat has nine calories per gram. I like walnuts and raisins as a snack. Healthy sounding isn't it. It also seems better than my fondness for cookies and candy. I especially like to put walnuts and raisins on my oatmeal that already has some raisins and walnuts, plus dates, in it.

Eight ounces is a cup. One ounce is one-eighth of a cup. If you have a one-eighth size measuring cup to look at, you might find it also has the words one oz printed on it. To me it looks so tiny compared to the hand full of nuts I used to drop on top of my cereal. The calories per one ounce serving for my walnuts are 190. The NF label also states that 160 of those calories are from fat.

Well nuts. Who knew? Darn that NF label. In the 190 calories, there is also four grams of protein (16 calories), two grams of fiber, and less than one gram of sugar with zero sodium. But my total fat for that little bitty bunch of nuts is 18 grams (162 calories). Now like the potato chips, I can incorporate this into my Daily Nutrition Spreadsheet and come out close enough to the DGA. So all is not lost, it is just acknowledged and put into perspective for being able to have some of my comfort foods that day.

Chapter 7

Targeting a Nutrition

Let's say you wake up one morning and decide you aren't getting enough fiber in your diet. (Sounds like a commercial doesn't it.) So you go get your Daily Nutrition Spreadsheet and start looking in your kitchen cabinets and refrigerator to see what you can eat that day to meet your fiber needs within your calorie level.

That's what I did one day and I was surprised how well I did on the other nutrition needs when I wrote it all down in the DNS. As always, my sugar grams were a pain to look at but the fat and cholesterol were real good. As usual, I didn't hit my potassium levels but I rationalized that since companies don't have to add that, I hoped I came closer than what it said on the DNS.

I'm going to show you what I had for breakfast, lunch, and dinner with a snack that day. It's going to sound pretty good on paper. But after I analyzed it, I wondered if I should have eliminated the walnuts I ate that had 190 calories for one-eighth of a cup and instead, replaced it with a second cup of soup at lunch for 110 calories. It would have been much more filling and it had three grams of fiber compared to the walnuts two grams of fiber. Oh well. Close enough. I do like my walnuts.

Breakfast: Coffee with sugar and creamer. One-half cup fruit, one packet of oatmeal, added one-eighth cup walnuts and one-fourth cup raisins.

Lunch: One cup soup, four club crackers, one-half cup fruit.

Dinner: Tuna, (I added salt) and light Mayonnaise on two slices of whole wheat bread. One cup skim milk and one-half cup mixed vegetables.

Snack   Three golden Oreo cookies.

Total Calories 1,480 at the 1,500 caloric level.

For a better look at how I did that day, in the first column below, I listed the nutrients on the DNS. Next to that I listed the amount of grams, milligrams, and percentages needed to meet the 1,500 calorie level of nutrients. Then I put the amount of total nutrients I ate by each one. Last, I put the difference that happened as a plus or a minus of the nutrient needed and you'll see they were fine except for potassium which is never good, but I keep trying.

	NF Label	Actual	Results	
Calories	1500	1480	-20	good
Total Fat	48 gm	31	-17	good
Cholesterol	300 mg	49	-251	good
Sodium	2400 mg	2410	+10	good
Carbohydrates	225 gm	217	-8	good
Fiber	19 mg	19		good
Protein	38 gm	41	+3	good

Potassium	2625 mg	1507	-1118	not so good
Sugar	not given but 122 gm @ 4 grams X 15 calories = 457 calories			

My added sugar for coffee was four teaspoons which equaled 60 calories. So it looks like the other food's natural and added sugar grams are why the sugar total came to 457 calories. The tropical fruit had 14 grams, raisins had 29, applesauce 19, milk and oatmeal came in at 11. Each cookie was only 6 grams. Sugar sucks.

The other foods had zero sugar (think walnuts at 190 calories) or were less than seven grams. I don't want to give up fruit and milk. The oatmeal came with raisins, dates, and walnuts and so the plain oatmeal probably would have had fewer sugar grams in it. So as it turns out, almost one-third of the calories I ate that day came from sugar (1480 divided by 3 = 493). And even worse, I only added 16 grams of sugar which came to just 60 calories meaning added sugars came to 397 calories.

So if you need to watch your sugar intake because you have to, or you want to, using the Daily Nutrition Spreadsheet is one way to do it.

As for the vitamins, calcium and iron, the percentage for them at a 1,500 calorie level is 75%. But the Nutrition Facts label percentage information is based on the 2,000 calorie level to reach their 100% for the Dietary Guidelines for Americans. Just those last two sentences sent my poor math skills into a nosedive. So since I have to use the NF 100 percent, and if I reach 75%, I like to think I've met the needed level for the day.

Vitamin A came to 115%, well over the amount for 2,000 calories. I have found that it is the easiest vitamin to meet. Vitamin C came to 57% and Vitamin D (that I track for myself) came to 40% which was from the milk and tuna. My calcium at 50% and the iron at 43% came in low which is why I take supplements for them and Vitamin D. I've noticed that my Vitamin C evens out over the week of food and so I don't worry about it too much.

A copy of the Daily Nutrition Spreadsheet I used, (DNS 16—Judy's Food Day), is in the back of the book so you can see how it all played out according to what this average Judy understands from the 2005 and 2010 Dietary Guidelines for Americans. I've also included another spreadsheet with the average food costs that day, where I was able to have cookies with my ice cream (DNS 17—$5 Average Food Cost at 1,500 Calorie Level). Once more, I can't urge you enough to please read these two Guidelines yourself, for yourself, to check the information that may be directed to you and your needs.

Chapter 8

A Bit About Vegan Vittles

Vegans and adults who are over 50 years old, who are not vegans, do have something in common. Vitamin B12. The 2010 Dietary Guidelines for Americans encourage these two groups to be sure they have an adequate daily amount of this vitamin through fortified foods or by taking dietary supplements. The only nutrient of concern that the DGA mentions for vegans is about protein foods. Unlike the lacto-ovo vegetarians who do consume milk and eggs that contain protein, vegans do not consume any animal products. They rely on plants (vegetables), nuts, seeds, and soy products for their protein.

I discovered that green beans, the ones that have the string running down the middle, and green peas are not a good plant source for protein. The green beans have a minimal amount of protein listed on the Nutrition Facts label, usually at one gram. They belong with the onions, lettuce, and celery group due to similar nutrient content. The green peas are considered a starchy vegetable and they are put in that group even though they have up to four grams of protein listed on the NF label. The protein peas are split peas and black-eyed peas plus garbanzo beans which are also know as chickpeas.

For vegans, the supply of plant foods with protein is vegetables like red kidney beans, pinto beans, black beans, navy beans, and lentils. There is also protein in what I call tree foods which are high in calories. These are nuts like pecans, almonds, walnuts, and macadamia. Peanuts are actually legumes that grow under the ground like potatoes. One of our presidents was a peanut farmer.

Seeds, like sunflower and pumpkin, are also high in calories. The processed soybean products are numerous, like milk, cheese, yogurt, and of course tofu. Soybean products are also added to foods like baked goods. The DGA mentioned rice milk as being a calcium-fortified beverage.

I did find some powdered soy protein mix with several grams of protein. The Nutrition Facts label did not show milk as an ingredient but the package had a statement at the bottom of the label that it contained milk ingredients. The powdered whey protein mix had the same statement. Both protein mixes were marketed as a protein powder. I didn't use either in my Daily Nutrition Spreadsheet.

Although dairy products are not eaten by vegans, there are calcium alternatives. So there are many calcium-fortified foods that can be consumed to meet the Daily Value for this mineral. I buy orange juice that is fortified with calcium and vitamin D to help me ensure I meet my Daily Value. Soymilk and some cereals are fortified with calcium.

When I started making out a DNS with vegan nutrient needs in mind, I found that the best way was the same way I started making out the original DNS spreadsheet. First I needed the Nutrition Facts label information off of the foods that I needed to exchange for dairy and animal protein. After I had gathered a few of them, I was ready to add them into the regular Daily Nutrition Spreadsheets as needed. (DNS 15—Vegan Labels)

I used the 2,000 calorie level DNS and decided on the breakfast items from my list first. They were a cup of raisin bran cereal with a cup of soy milk and then an apple. For lunch I listed a veggie Griller pattie with vegan cheese and a one-half cup of canned peas. Then I added some peanut butter on whole wheat bread to eat then or later on as a snack.

For dinner I added a veggie Turk'y pattie with a slice of whole wheat bread, a sweet potato and baked beans to have with my cup of soymilk. For a snack in the afternoon I put down a cup of orange juice, squeezed from fresh oranges, and fortified with calcium and vitamin D.

For the evening snack I listed soy ice cream topped with 1/4 cup of raisins. The total calories came to 2,042. There were zero milligrams of cholesterol. The potassium came to 3,233 of the needed 3,500 milligrams. The calcium came to 165% of the 100% Daily Value and the protein was 78 grams of the needed 50 grams.

As to the sugar and fats that the DGA is always concerned about, the total grams for sugar came to 127. Sugar is a carbohydrate and it has four calories per gram. So that's 508 calories. The total grams of fat came to 70. Fat has nine calories per gram. So that's 630 calories. I can see why they are concerned. As a matter of further information for your calculations, protein has four calories per gram.

All of this was laid out without me giving any thought about what foods I needed on there before I listed them. That's how helpful it can be to have a spreadsheet with all of the label information from what you usually eat completed first. Then it's just a matter of listing what you want to eat for breakfast, lunch, dinner, and snacks. After you see the totals for each nutrient, you can adjust as needed.

I didn't adjust any item on my list ahead of time. The fat grams came to 70 of the intended 65, the sodium milligrams went just over the less than 2,400 at 2,635, and the carbohydrate grams were 258 of the planned 300. I had 54 milligrams of fiber which was twice the amount needed to meet the 25, in addition to going higher than the listed protein grams and calcium percentage. These items could easily be adjusted by checking for different foods from the spreadsheet that had the label information, and replace them. Using this method, I would come close enough to eating nutritiously using the Dietary Guidelines for Americans and still enjoy the way this average Judy likes to eat.

Vitamin A on the DNS showed it at 171%. Vitamin C was also over at 182% and vitamin D was 85%. Iron came in at 102%. The Daily Values to meet for the vitamins and minerals on the 2,000 calorie level is 100% (DNS 18—Vegan's Food Day).

Although I'm not a vegetarian or a vegan, it didn't seem very difficult to plan around the animal products because of the information on the Nutrition Facts label and putting it into the DNS. There were many other foods on my spreadsheet of label information that I didn't use which would help to make a very nice variety of menus over the week to eat like a vegan.

CHAPTER 9

The Nutrient Dense Thing

To get the most satisfaction for the fewest calories is really what the nutrient dense thing is about. Its food that's prepared without added solid fats, sugars, starches, and sodium as much as possible. It helps those who want to create a plan on how to fill up with a lot of food without the excess calories moving their weight up the scale. It's like getting the biggest bang for your nutrition buck. It's like hold the sugar and fats please because I want that second slice of watermelon or another handful of grapes.

However, for the average Judy it would be a couple of cookies or a candy bar because of those discretionary calorie allowances that the 2005 Dietary Guidelines for Americans mentioned in Table 1, at the bottom of page 10. It talks about when you have consumed the nutrient dense foods from all of the food groups, there may be some remaining calories left for that day at your calorie level. (The 2010 DGA uses SoFAS instead of discretionary calorie allowance. It stands for Solid Fats Added Sugars.)

Said another way, choosing low fat (skim milk) and low sugar (don't add any) foods from each food group, you will likely eat all of your nutrition requirements (grams/milligrams) at your chosen calorie level and still have some calories left over to consume at your discretion. The 2005 DGA even has the number of calories figured out for you at different calorie levels on page 53 in Appendix A-2 USDA Food Guide. It shows that at the 2,000 calorie level, you could have 267 calories left if you have chosen your nutrient dense foods wisely.

There is an example in Appendix A-3 on page 55 that shows the grams of solid fats and added sugars remaining to be used at the 2,000 calorie level. It is 18 grams of solid fat and 32 grams (8 tsp) of sugar. I can't see too many people looking at their spreadsheet to see what foods would meet those criteria to stay around the 267 calories. I automatically know that my two cookies and 3 pieces of candy come to 282 calories and that's how I would use those calories at my discretion. I would say those extra 15 calories were close enough to the way I try to eat nutritiously using the Dietary Guidelines for Americans.

That is really what the 2005 and 2010 Dietary Guidelines for Americans are about. Helping us make better decisions on how we eat depending on our health needs and how we want to eat given our particular circumstances. It's all there and has been since first published in 1980 and every five years since. Whether it's information about the specific population groups, food safety principles, or the food patterns from the USDA, DASH or vegan and vegetarian choices, they are based on scientific findings and we can choose to use them. I choose to eat as healthy as I can, using their information, to come close enough to the DGA and still enjoy eating.

―――≈∞∞∞≈―――

Nutrient dense food includes a variety of calories from all of the food groups. It's not about focusing on just some of the food groups like fruits and vegetables. There is a certain amount of energy from all of the foods we eat during our day that is used up (expended). If they are not used up, the calories are stored in the body. We don't get to choose where it's stored. So I guess it's true, we can't fool Mother Nature.

The science based information in the DGAs are the recommended amounts of nutrients we need depending on whether we are in one of the specific population groups or the average healthy adult. We eat food (calories) in order for it to be turned into energy that our bodies can use to get us through the day. Eating nutrient dense foods ensure we have that energy to use. I could eat my 1,200 to 1,500 calories a day in ice cream and still stay the same weight. I lived on snack food in the 1980's and stayed the same weight. That's not the point.

I had concerns about diabetes because my aunt on my father's side had it. Her son now has it. My parents were very concerned when I was a teenager that I might develop it. I was a soda jerk at our town's Rexall Drug store and ate my way through a lot of sweets. Just because I didn't develop it, I feel I may still have the potential. However, it was my cholesterol level that put me on the trail of how to change my eating habits to combat it. My husband had died young from three clogged arteries in his heart.

So, with these incentives in mind, I began to try to watch my food intake. At the time the only thing available was the doctors telling me to stop eating organ meats and of course eggs and a few other things that were known to have a high level of cholesterol in them. Then they came out with having people take a massive amount of Niacin. A guy in the office took that but it turned him red and made him hot at unexpected times. So I didn't try that.

Instead I developed my own eating plan like Quaker Puffed Wheat with skim milk and grapefruit in the mornings. I brought my total cholesterol down over 50 points which was closer to the total of 250 that was recommended at the time. Now I believe it's recommended to be 200 or below. Later the statin cholesterol lowering drugs were developed, and I went through four kinds and couldn't take any of them. But it turns out I have such a high HDL level which is a good thing, and my risk ratio is very low, also a good thing, that my concerns have lessen some about clogged arteries.

Finally, in the early 1990s, I noticed some information on a label that was on my can of vegetables. It was called the Nutrition Facts label.

I've been using it ever since. That's all I had to use at the time because I still had not heard of the Dietary Guidelines for Americans. I had already started my Daily Nutrition Spreadsheet when I came across the online version of the 2005 DGA. My knowledge increased and the nutrient dense thing became part of my daily eating habits.

Using my DNS has kept me on track to eat a good amount of my food in its nutrient dense form. I had been drinking skim milk since the 1980s, more fruits and vegetables when I had the Nutrition Facts label information, and then quit going through a fast food drive through restaurant every single day. I really like restaurants that are showing the nutrient information in their food now. And I really like knowing the amount of fats and sugars I'm eating each day so I can decease them if necessary and increase my nutrient dense foods accordingly.

⟞⟜⟝

Nutrient dense foods are fairly easy to spot. Think 90% lean ground beef instead of 75% or baked, skinless chicken breast compared to fried chicken. Look for cereal without added sugars by looking at the sugar grams on the NF label. When you look for applesauce, think about buying the unsweetened one, and you could choose the skim or 1% milk instead of whole milk. What this does is not add unnecessary calories to your food and makes it healthier for those who need to watch for this.

Following is a two day nutrient dense eating pattern for you to visually see what this can mean.

Breakfast   Whole grain toast topped with cinnamon and honey, banana, coffee, water.

Lunch   Lowfat vanilla yogurt topped with blueberries and strawberries (frozen/thawed, no sugar added) and 1 graham cracker.

Snack   One slice lowfat cheddar cheese and apple.

Dinner	Grilled boneless/skinless chicken breast, potatoes augratin, steamed broccoli, watermelon.
Breakfast	Bowl of cereal with skim milk, sliced banana, coffee, water.
Lunch	Tuna salad (made with light miracle whip and grapes), spinach in a low carb wrap.
Snack	Pretzels with a wedge of low fat Swiss cheese.
Dinner	Grilled salmon, baked potato, salad, grapes.

I did find a government online piece of information with the nutrition facts about raw food. I think it would help a lot in choosing nutrient dense food without the addition of fats and sugars. To get to the page I found, go to www.fda.gov. There are tabs across the top to click and I clicked on the second tab to the right labeled food. Then at the top right of the page that came up is a white search box that you can type in the words, raw vegetable poster. Up comes one more example of our tax dollars being put to good use. It's an amazing amount of information on vegetables like my Daily Nutrition Spreadsheet has.

Then if you will look around at the top area of that web page, you will see at the left, a link to click on that says nutrition information for raw fruits, vegetables, and fish. They are very small and you will need to click on one of the PDFs to the right of them to print it out. I chose the small PDF. There's lots of great information there too. Good luck.

So there you have it. The nutrient dense thing explained by the average Judy trying to understand all of the information in the Dietary Guidelines for Americans, and how I tried to understand the Nutrition Facts label for its information, and then apply all of it to what I eat.

I want to wish all the best to you on finding your own path to a healthy eating pattern.

Total Daily Nutrition Based on 1000 Calories Cholesterol & Sodium same all calorie levels.	Serving Size or Amount	Calories 35gm Total Fat	<300mg Total Cholesterol	<2400mg Sodium	150gm Carbs	15mg Fiber	25gm Protein	1750mg Potassium	Sugar grams	5000IU Vit A	60mg Vit C	1000mg Calcium	18mg Iron	400IU Vit D	$0.00 Average Cost Per Serving
		0	0	0	0	0	0	0	0	0	0	0	0	0	0

Percent totals at the top of these columns are for the 100% on the NF label needed at 2,000 calories

DNS 1—1,000 Calorie Level

Total Daily Nutrition Based on 1500 Calories Cholesterol & Sodium same all calorie levels	Serving Size or Amount	Calories Total	50gm Total Fat	<300mg Choles-terol	<2400mg Sodium	225gm Carbs	20mg Fiber	38gm Protein	2625mg Potas-sium	Sugar grams	5000IU Vit A	60mg Vit C	1000mg Calcium	18mg Iron	400IU Vit D	$0.00 Average Cost Per Serving
		0	0	0	0	0	0	0	0	0	0	0	0	0	0	

Percent totals at the top of these columns are for the 100% on the NF label needed at 2,000 calories

DNS 2—1,500 Calorie Level

Total Daily Nutrition			0	0	0	0	0	0	0	0	0	0	0	0	0	$0.00
Based on 2000 Calories	Serving	Calories	65 gm	<300mg	<2400mg	300gm	25 mg	50gm	3500mg	grams	5000IU	60mg	1000mg	18mg	400IU	Average
Cholesterol & Sodium	Size or	Total	Total	Choles-	Sodium	Carbs	Fiber	Protein	Potas-	Sugar	Vit A	Vit C	Calcium	Iron	Vit D	Cost Per
same all calorie levels	Amount		Fat	terol					sium		Percent totals at the top of these columns are for the 100% on the NF label needed at 2,000 calories					Serving

DNS 3—2,000 Calorie Level

Total Daily Nutrition Based on 2500 Calories Cholesterol & Sodium same all calorie levels.	Serving Size or Amount	Calories	80gm Total Fat	<300mg Choles-terol	<2400mg Sodium	375gm Carbs	30mg Fiber	63gm Protein	4375mg Potas-sium	Sugar grams	5000IU Vit A	60mg Vit C	1000mg Calcium	18mg Iron	400IU Vit D	$0.00 Average Cost Per Serving
		0	0	0	0	0	0	0	0	0	0	0	0	0	0	
											Percent totals at the top of these columns are for the 100% on the NF label needed at 2,000 calories					

DNS 4—2,500 Calorie Level

Total Daily Nutrition	Serving	Calories	Total Fat	Cholesterol	Sodium	Carbs	Fiber	Protein	Potassium	Sugar grams	Vit A	Vit C	Calcium	Iron	Vit D	Average Cost Per Serving
Based on **3000** Calories		0	95gm 0	<300mg 0	<2400mg 0	450gm 0	35 mg 0	75gm 0	5250mg 0	0	5000IU 0	60mg 0	1000mg 0	18mg 0	400IU 0	$0.00
Cholesterol & Sodium	Size or	Total	Total Fat	Choles- terol	Sodium	Carbs	Fiber	Protein	Potas- sium	grams	Vit A	Vit C	Calcium	Iron	Vit D	Cost Per
same all calorie levels.	Amount									Percent totals at the top of these columns are for the 100% on the NF label needed at 2,000						Serving

DNS 5—3,000 Calorie Level

GRAINS	Ser Size	Total Calories	Total Fat	Choles- terol	Sodium	Carbs	Fiber	Protein	Potas- sium	Sugar	Vit A 100%	Vit C 100%	Calcium 100%	Iron 100%	Vit D 100%
Cholesterol & Sodium levels remain the same no matter what the calorie level			I round the numbers - such as <.5 will be 0, but .5 will be 1								% based on 2,000 calorie level				
Bread, Mrs Bairds 100% whole wheat	1 Slice	60	1	0	110	12	2	3	0	2	0	0	4	4	0
Bread, Mrs Bairds double fiber whole grains	1 Slice	60	0	0	110	13	5	3	0	2	0	0	10	6	0
Cereal bar, Nutri-grain Apple Cinnamon	1 bar	120	3	0	110	24	3	2	0	12	15	0	20	10	0
Cereal, Cheerios apple cinnamon	3/4 C	120	2	0	115	24	2	2	65	10	10	10	10	25	10
Cereal, Cheerios frosted	3/4 C	110	1	0	170	23	2	2	55	10	10	10	10	25	10
Cereal, Fiber One honey squares	3/4 C	80	1	0	140	25	10	1	70	3	10	10	40	25	0
Cereal, Kellogg's frosted flakes single serving	1 Box	130	0	0	160	30	1	2	0	12	10	10	0	25	0
Cereal, Quaker Oats, Raisin, Dates, Walnuts	1 pkt	140	3	0	190	27	3	3	140	11	20	0	10	20	0
Cereal, Raisin Bran	1 C	190	1	0	210	46	7	5	390	18	10	0	2	25	0
Crackers, Keebler Club crackers	4 crkrs	70	3	0	125	9	2	1	0	1	0	0	0	0	0
Pasta, Knorr bettuccini butter & herb	2/3 C	220	3	5	530	40	2	7	0	4	0	0	4	10	0
Pasta, Knorr shells in garlic cheese sauce	2/3 C	250	5	10	560	43	2	8	0	3	2	0	4	10	0
Popcorn, Orville Redenbacker's	4 C	170	14	0	330	14	3	2	0	0	0	0	0	2	0
Rice, Knorr rice sides, creamy chicken	1/2 C	250	2	0	750	51	1	7	0	3	8	2	4	15	0
Rice, Minute brown wild	1 C	230	5	0	130	42	5	5	135	0	0	0	0	4	0

DNS 6—Grain Labels

VEGETABLES	Ser Size	Total Calories	Total Fat	Choles-terol	Sodium	Carbs	Fiber	Protein	Potas-sium	Sugar	Vit A	Vit C	Calcium	Iron	Vit D
Cholesterol & Sodium levels remain the same no matter what the calorie level			I round the numbers - such as <.5 will be 0, but .5 will be 1								% based on 2,000 calorie level	100%	100%	100%	100%
											100%				
Asparagus, Green Giant cut spears	1/2 C	20	0	0	420	3	1	2		1	6	15	0	2	0
Beans, Bush's navy	1/2 C	80	0	0	470	17	7	6	290	0	0	0	4	10	0
Beans, Del Monte lima	1/2 C	80	0	0	390	15	4	4	0	0	2	8	2	8	0
Beans, Green Giant green, 50% less sodium	1/2 C	20	0	0	200	4	1	1	0	2	6	4	2	2	0
Beans, S&W butter	1/2 C	80	0	0	500	19	5	6	0	0	0	4	6	10	0
Beans, VanCamp's Pork & Beans	1/2 C	110	1	0	420	23	6	6	0	7	0	0	4	10	0
Beets, Best Choice sliced beets	1/2 C	40	0	0	350	8	1	1	0	6	0	0	1	1	0
Carrots, Del Monte	1/2 C	35	0	0	300	8	3	0	0	5	300	6	2	2	0
Corn, Del Monte whole kernel corn no salt added	1/2 C	60	1	0	10	11	3	2	0	7	0	6	0	2	0
Corn, Fritos corn chips original 2 oz	1 Pkg	320	20	0	320	32	3	3	0	0	0	0	4	2	0
Greens, Bush's turnip & mustard greens	1/2 C	25	0	0	300	3	2	2	0	1	70	15	10	6	0
Hominy, Bush's golden hominy	1/2 C	60	0	0	550	13	3	1	0	0	4	2	2	2	0
Mixed - Frozen, Birds Eye, Broccoli Cauliflower and Carrots	3/4 C	30	0	0	30	5	2	1	0	2	15	30	2	2	0
Mixed, Green Giant carrots, green beans, sweet peas, corn, lima beans	1/2 C	45	0	0	260	10	2	2	200	3	50	2	0	2	0
Peas, Libby's Naturals sweet peas	1/2 C	60	0	0	15	10	3	4	0	5	6	20	2	8	0
Potato, Del Monte whole new potatoes	2 Med	60	0	0	280	13	2	1	300	0	0	15	2	2	0
Potato, Lays classic potato chips	1 Oz	160	10	0	170	15	1	2	350	0	0	10	0	2	0
Potato, sweet raw 5 oz	1 Med	100	0	0	70	23	4	2	440	7	120	30	4	4	0
Potato, white raw 5 oz	1 Med	110	0	0	0	9	2	3	620	1	0	45	2	6	0
Spinach, Allens Popeye	1/2 C	45	1	0	35	4	3	2	0	0	160	25	15	15	0
Yams, Princella sweet potatoes in light syrup	1/2 C	160	0	0	35	39	3	0	0	20	220	8	2	8	0

DNS 7—Vegetable Labels

FRUIT Cholesterol & Sodium levels remain the same no matter what the calorie level	Ser Size	Total Calories	Total Fat	Choles-terol	Sodium	Carbs	Fiber	Protein	Potas-sium	Sugar	Vit A 100%	Vit C 100%	Calcium 100%	Iron 100%	Vit D 100%
			I round the numbers - such as <.5 will be 0, but .5 will be 1								% based on 2,000 calorie level				
Apple, Luck's fried with cinnamon	1/2 C	100	0	0	30	25	2	0	0	17	0	20	0	0	0
Apple, Musselman's chunky applesauce 100% American grown apples	1/2 C	90	0	0	10	23	2	0	0	19	0	0	0	0	0
Apple, raw 2 3/4" with skin	1 Med	72	0	0	0	19	4	4	148	14	15	10	8	0	0
Apricot, Del Monte unpeeled in light syrup	1/2 C	80	0	0	10	21	1	0	0	20	30	100	0	2	0
Banana	1 Med	105	26	3	0	26	3	2	422	14	2	10	0	1	0
Grapefruit, Del Monte red, in light syrup	1/2 C	90	0	0	0	21	1	1	0	17	0	100	2	15	0
Grapefruit, Del Monte red, no sugar added	1/2 C	40	0	0	15	10	0	0	110	6	10	100	0	0	0
Juice, Dole tropical fruit 100%	1/2 C	60	0	0	5	15	1	0	160	14	10	45	0	0	0
Juice, Old Orchard 100% grape juice	1 C	160	0	0	20	41	0	0	0	39	0	130	0	0	0
Juice, Florida's 100% squeezed from fresh oranges with calcium & vitamin D	1 C	110	0	0	0	26	0	2	450	22	0	120	35	0	25
Juice, Tree Top apple from concentrate	1 C	120	0	0	25	29	0	0	280	26	0	120	0	0	0
Juice, Welch's white grape peach 100% juice no added sugars	1 C	140	0	0	20	36	0	0	0	35	0	100	0	0	0
Orange, Del Monte Mandarin in light syrup	1/2 C	70	0	0	10	17	0	0	90	17	0	100	0	0	0
Orange, Dole Mandarin in light syrup	1/2 C	80	0	0	5	19	0	0	55	18	10	50	0	0	0
Orange, Roland Mandarin in water	1/2 C	45	0	0	15	10	1	1	0	7	8	25	6	2	0
Peach, Del Monte sliced peaches	1/2 C	50	0	0	10	14	2	1	0	12	6	8	0	2	0
Peach, Doles diced peaches in 100% juice	1/2 C	80	0	0	5	19	1	0	90	18	4	45	0	0	0
Pear, Del Monte sliced in heavy syrup	1/2 C	100	0	0	10	24	1	0	0	23	0	4	0	0	0
Pear, Libby's halves in heavy syrup	1/2 C	100	0	0	10	25	2	0	80	19	0	0	0	0	0
Pineapple, Best Choice sliced	3 Slices	70	0	0	10	17	1	0	0	14	0	2	2	2	0
Raisins, Sun-Maid regular & golden raisins	1/4 C	130	0	0	10	31	2	1	310	29	0	0	2	6	0

DNS 8—Fruit Labels

DAIRY, etc.

Cholesterol & Sodium levels remain the same no matter what the calorie level

I round the numbers - such as <.5 will be 0, but .5 will be 1

% based on 2,000 calorie level

	Ser Size	Total Calories	Total Fat	Choles-terol	Sodium	Carbs	Fiber	Protein	Potas-sium	Sugar	Vit A 100%	Vit C 100%	Calcium 100%	Iron 100%	Vit D 100%
Cheese, Alma Creamery sharp cheddar	1 Oz	110	9	30	170	0	0	7	0	0	6	0	20	2	0
Cheese, cottage, A&E 4% milkfat small curd	1/2 C	110	5	20	460	3	0	12	0	3	4	0	8	2	0
Cheese, Kraft American Singles	1 Slice	70	5	15	220	2	0	4	0	1	4	0	25	0	10
Cheese, Kraft sharp cheddar cubes	7 pcs	120	10	30	200	0	0	7	0	0	8	0	20	0	0
Cheese, Wisconsin sharp cheddar	1 Oz	110	9	30	180	0	0	6	0	0	8	0	20	0	0
Milk, Horizon organic, fat-free 32 mg Omega-3	1 Cup	90	0	5	135	13	0	9	420	12	10	10	30	0	25
Milk, Roberts skim milk, Vit A&D, fat-free	1 Cup	80	0	5	120	11	0	8	0	11	10	2	30	0	25
Vitamins, Centrum Silver chewable	1 Tblt	5	0	0	0	2					80	125	20	0	0
Vitamins, Viactiv	1 Chew	20	0	0	0	0	0	0	0	3	0	0	50	0	125
Yogurt, Chobani Greek peach	6 Oz	140	0	0	65	20	0	14	0	19	2	2	20	10	0
Yogurt, Dannon 99% fat free peach	1 cntnr	110	1	5	65	20	0	5	220	19	0	0	15	0	0
Yogurt, Oikos Organic Greek non-fat honey	1/2 C	90	0	0	40	13	0	10	0	13	0	0	10	0	0

DNS 9—Dairy Labels

PROTEIN	Ser	Total	Total	Choles-	Sodium	Carbs	Fiber	Protein	Potas-	Sugar	Vit A	Vit C	Calcium	Iron	Vit D
Cholesterol & Sodium levels remain the same no matter what the calorie level	Size	Calories	Fat	terol					sium		100%	100%	100%	100%	100%
			I round the numbers - such as <.5 will be 0, but .5 will be 1								% based on 2,000 calorie level				
Beef, ground round, 86% lean	4 oz	230	16	75	0	0	0	21	0	0	0	0	0	15	0
Beef, Hormel beef roast au jus	5 Oz	210	10	80	450	3	0	28	0	3	0	0	0	10	0
Beef, Hormel meat loaf with tomato sauce	5 Oz	260	13	60	850	13	1	22	0	7	2	0	4	10	0
Chicken, Boars Head EverRoast breast	2 Oz	50	0	30	440	1	0	13	160	1	0	2	0	2	0
Chicken, Hormel canned chunk in water	2 Oz	60	3	25	250	0	0	9	0	0	0	0	0	2	0
Chicken, Libby's Vienna sausage	3 Links	100	8	50	410	1	0	5	0	0	0	0	2	2	0
Chicken, Oscar Mayer cooked deli meat	2 Oz	60	2	30	710	1	0	10	0	0	0	0	0	4	0
Chicken, Swanson chicken breast in water	2 Oz	50	1	20	270	1	0	10	0	1	0	0	0	0	
Chicken, Tyson chicken breast in water	2 Oz	60	1	30	200	0	0	13	0	0	0	0	0	2	0
Egg, Egglands hard cooked, vegetarian fed	1 Egg	60	4	160	55	0	0	5	0	0	6	0	2	4	20
Egg, Egglands large brown vegetarian fed cage free organic, 100mg of Omega 3	1 Egg	70	4	170	65	0	0	6	0	0	10	0	2	4	20
Egg, Land of Lakes large white all-natural vegetarian fed, 350 mg Omega-3	1 Egg	70	5	215	65	1	0	6	0	0	6	0	2	4	0
Hot Dog, Ball Park beef	1 Frank	150	13	30	440	3	0	5	280	2	0	4	0	2	0
Nuts, Planters Walnuts	1 Oz	190	18	0	0	4	2	4	125	0	0	0	2	4	0
Peanut Butter, Skippy creamy	2 Tbsp	190	16	0	150	7	2	7	0	3	0	0	0	4	0
Peanut Butter, Skippy natural super chunk	2 Tbsp	190	17	0	125	6	2	7	0	3	0	0	0	4	0
Salmon, Bumble Bee wild Alaska 2.2 oz	1/4 C	100	5	40	220	0	0	13	220	0	4	0	30	4	0
Salmon, Chicken of the Sea pink in water	2 Oz	60	2	20	280	0	0	10	0	0	0	0	0	4	0
Spam, Hormel Foods	2 Oz	180	16	40	790	1	0	7	0	0	0	0	0	2	0
Tuna, Starkist Albacore white in water 2.6 oz	1 Pkt	90	2	30	310	1	1	18	240	0	0	0	0	2	20
Turkey, Hormel canned chunk in water	2 Oz	60	2	30	280	1	0	9	0	0	0	0	0	2	0

DNS 10—Protein Labels

OILS FATS SNACKS

OILS FATS SNACKS	Ser Size	Total Calories	Total Fat	Choles-terol	Sodium	Carbs	Fiber	Protein	Potas-sium	Sugar	Vit A 100%	Vit C 100%	Calcium 100%	Iron 100%	Vit D 100%
Cholesterol & Sodium levels remain the same no matter what the calorie level			I round the numbers - such as <.5 will be 0, but .5 will be 1	terol					sium			% based on 2,000 calorie level			
Butter, Best Choice butter	1 Tbsp	100	11	30	90	0	0	0	0	0	8	0	0	0	0
Butter, Land O Lakes butter	1 Tbsp	100	11	30	0	0	0	0	0	0	8	0	0	0	0
Butter, Land O Lakes spread	1 Tbsp	70	8	0	80	0	0	0	0	0	10	0	0	0	0
Butter, Parkay original spread	1 Tbsp	60	7	0	90	0	0	0	0	0	10	0	0	0	0
Butter, Parkay stick	1 Tbsp	90	10	0	105	0	0	0	0	0	10	0	0	0	0
Butter, Promise 60% vegetable oil spread	1 Tbsp	80	8	0	85	0	0	0	0	0	10	0	0	0	15
Candy, Hershey snack size bar	3 Bars	200	12	10	35	25	1	3	0	23	0	0	8	2	0
Candy, Milky Way fun size	2 Bars	150	6	5	55	24	0	1	0	20	0	0	4	0	0
Candy, Queen Anne chocolate covered cherries	2 pcs	150	4	0	10	30	0	0	0	26	0	0	2	2	0
Candy, Reeses miniatures peanut butter cup	5 pcs	210	12	4	115	22	1	4	0	19	0	0	2	2	0
Candy, Rolo chocolate caramel	7 pcs	190	8	5	75	27	0	2	0	25	4	0	0	0	0
Cookies, Keebler sandies cashew	2 Cks	160	9	4	110	18	0	2	0	7	0	0	0	4	0
Cookies, Oreo golden double stuf	2 Cks	150	7	0	80	21	0	0	15	12	0	0	0	2	0
Ice Cream, Blue Bell cherry vanilla	1/2 C	150	7	30	50	19	0	3	0	16	6	0	10	2	0
Ice Cream, Edys Turtles	1/2 C	160	9	25	50	18	0	3	0	14	8	0	6	0	0
Jelly/Jam, Smucker's strawberry jam seedless	1 Tbsp	50	0	0	0	13	0	0	0	12	0	0	0	0	0
Olives, Lindsay Spanish manzanilla stuffed	5 Olives	25	3	0	240	0	0	0	0	0	0	0	0	0	0
Pickles, Vlasic sweet midgets	1 Oz	30	0	0	170	7	0	0	0	7	0	0	0	0	0
Salad Dressing, Dorothy Lynch fat free	1 Tbsp	30	0	0	80	7	0	0	0	7	0	0	0	0	0
Salad Dressing, Hellimans mayonnaise light	1 Tbsp	35	4	4	125	0	0	0	0	0	0	0	0	0	0
Sugar, C&H granulated white 4 grams. 50 grams equals 10% of the 2,000 calorie level	1 tsp	15	0	0	0	4	0	0	0	0	0	0	0	0	0

DNS 11—SoFAS (Oils, Fats, Snacks) Labels

CANNED MEALS	Ser Size	Total Calories	Total Fat	Choles-terol	Sodium	Carbs	Fiber	Protein	Potas-sium	Sugar	Vit A 100%	Vit C 100%	Calcium 100%	Iron 100%	Vit D 100%
Cholesterol & Sodium levels remain the same no matter what the calorie level			**I round the numbers – such as <.5 will be 0, but .5 will be 1**								**% based on 2,000 calorie level**				
Soup, Campbells bean & ham & vegetables	1 Cup	180	2	10	780	30	8	11	0	5	50	0	6	10	0
Soup, Campbells Beef tips with veggies	1 Cup	110	1	15	790	18	3	7	0	4	20	2	2	6	0
Soup, Campbells Beef, noodle	1 Cup	120	2	20	670	17	3	8	650	6	50	2	6	8	0
Soup, Campbells Beef, veggies, Dumplings	1 Cup	130	2	25	800	20	3	8	320	8	20	2	2	6	0
Soup, Campbells chicken & egg noodles	1 Cup	100	3	15	480	13	2	7	700	1	20	0	2	2	0
Soup, Campbells chicken & vegetables	1 Cup	90	1	10	410	16	3	5	920	4	30	4	4	4	0
Soup, Campbells chicken & vegetables&pasta	1 Cup	110	2	15	890	15	2	8	0	3	50	0	2	4	0
Soup, Campbells chicken broccoli cheese with potato	1 Cup	210	11	20	880	20	3	7	0	6	20	6	2	0	0
Soup, Campbells chicken noodle	1 Cup	110	3	20	790	14	2	7	0	2	20	0	2	4	0
Soup, Campbells chicken noodle 30% less sodium + one can water	1/2 C	60	2	10	450	8	1	3	240	1	15	0	0	0	0
Soup, Campbells Chicken, with vegetables	1 Cup	110	2	15	710	17	3	6	0	3	25	2	2	4	0
Soup, Campbells salisbury steak	1 Cup	150	5	20	890	18	2	9	0	7	50	2	4	6	0
Soup, Campbells sirloin burger & vegetables	1 Cup	130	3	15	800	18	3	8	0	4	30	4	2	10	0
Soup, Campbells sirloin steak & vegetables	1 Cup	130	2	10	890	19	3	8	0	15	30	2	2	6	0
Soup, Campbells vegetable	1 Cup	120	1	0	410	24	4	3	1050	8	40	0	6	4	0
Soup, Campbells vegetable & pasta	1 Cup	130	2	4	930	23	3	4	0	9	60	4	4	6	0

DNS 12—Canned Meal Labels

FROZEN MEALS	Ser Size	Total Calories	Total Fat	Choles-terol	Sodium	Carbs	Fiber	Protein	Potas-sium	Sugar	Vit A	Vit C	Calcium	Iron	Vit D
Cholesterol & Sodium levels remain the same no matter what the caloric level			I round the numbers - such as <.5 will be 0, but .5 will be 1								100%	100%	100%	100%	100%
											% based on 2,000 calorie level				
Kid Cuisine, Chicken Breast Nuggets	1 pkg	430	18	25	50	54	6	14	550	12	15	0	8	10	0
Healthy Choice, Chicken Parmigiana	1 pkg	340	9	25	580	49	7	16	540	17	10	50	10	6	0
Healthy Choice, Honey Roasted Turkey	1 pkg	250	4	40	350	36	5	17	640	20	70	45	6	4	0
Healthy Choice, Oven Roasted Chicken	1 pkg	240	5	35	530	33	4	15	680	12	20	15	4	4	0
Healthy Choice, Salisbury Steak	1 pkg	320	7	35	590	45	8	18	790	18	6	80	10	10	0
Lean Cuisine, Baked Chicken	1 pkg	240	7	30	600	30	2	14	770	4	0	0	4	10	0
Lean Cuisine, Grilled Chicken Caesar	1 pkg	250	6	30	610	30	3	19	560	2	10	35	15	4	0
Lean Cuisine, Grilled Chicken Primavera	1 pkg	220	4	25	580	30	5	17	570	5	10	50	10	10	0
Lean Cuisine, Herb Roasted Chicken	1 pkg	180	4	30	490	20	5	16	890	5	6	40	6	4	0

DNS 13—Frozen Meal Labels

PACKAGED MEALS	Ser Size	Total Calories	Total Fat	Choles-terol	Sodium	Carbs	Fiber	Protein	Potas-sium	Sugar	Vit A	Vit C	Calcium	Iron	Vit D
Cholesterol & Sodium levels remain the same no matter what the calorie level				I round the numbers - such as <.5 will be 0, but .5 will be 1							100%	100%	100%	100%	100%
											% based on 2,000 calorie level				
Lunchables, bologna (chicken/pork) American cheese, crackers, cherry juice, Kit Kat	1 Pkg	300	16	45	510	32	1	10	0	19	4	8	20	15	0
Lunchables, ham, American cheese, crackers, cherry juice, fun size Butterfinger	1 Pkg	320	13	30	580	40	1	11	0	21	4	15	15	6	0
Lunchables, ham, swiss, crackers	1 Pkg	260	13	45	720	22	1	14	0	5	4	20	20	8	0
Lunchables, turkey, mozzarella cheese, crackers, punch, Reese's peanut butter cup	1 Pkg	300	12	20	530	38	1	12	0	26	0	80	20	6	0

DNS 14—Packaged Meal Labels

Vegan Variety Foods	Ser	Total	Total	Choles-	Sodium	Carbs	Fiber	Protein	Potas-	Sugar	Vit A	Vit C	Calcium	Iron	Vit D	Vit B12
Cholesterol & Sodium levels remain the same no matter what the calorie level	Size	Calories	Fat	terol					sium		100%	100%	100%	100%	100%	100%
			I round the numbers – such as <5 will be 0, but .5 will be 1								% based on 2,000 calorie level					
Beans - baked	1/2 C	150	1	0	530	30	8	6	390	8	0	2	6	10	0	0
Beans - dark red kidney	1/2 C	105	0	0	250	22	8	7	400	3	0	0	8	10	0	0
Beans - lima	1/2 C	100	0	0	330	19	8	6	410	1	2	2	6	10	0	8
Beans - navy	1/2 C	80	0	0	470	17	7	6	290	0	0	0	4	10	0	0
Bread - 100% whole wheat	1 Slice	60	1	0	110	12	2	3	0	2	0	0	4	4	0	0
Bread - cinnamon swirl bagel	1 Bgl	270	2	0	390	53	3	10	0	10	0	0	10	20	0	0
Cereal, Fiber One honey squares	3/4 C	80	1	0	140	25	10	1	70	3	10	10	40	25	0	25
Cereal, Raisin Bran	1 C	190	1	0	210	46	7	5	390	18	10	0	2	25	0	25
Cheese - vegan	1 Oz	90	7	0	260	7	1	1	0	0	0	0	0	0	0	0
Fruit - Apple, raw 2 3/4 " with skin	1 Med	72	0	0	0	19	4	4	148	14	15	10	8	0	0	0
Fruit - Banana	1 Med	105	26	3	0	26	3	2	422	14	2	10	0	1	0	0
Fruit - Juice, 100% squeezed from fresh oranges with calcium & vitamin D	1 C	110	0	0	0	26	0	2	450	22	0	120	35	0	25	0
Fruit - Raisins, regular & golden raisins	1/4 C	130	0	0	10	31	2	1	310	29	0	0	2	6	0	0
Nuts, Planters Walnuts	1 Oz	190	18	0	0	4	2	4	125	0	0	0	2	4	0	0
Peanut Butter, Skippy natural super chunk	2 Tbsp	190	17	0	125	6	2	7	0	3	0	0	0	4	0	0
Rice, Minute brown wild	1 C	230	5	0	130	42	5	5	135	0	0	0	0	4	0	0
Soy Ice Cream	1 C	400	18	0	0	0	10	4	0	0	0	0	0	0	0	0
Soy Milk,	1 C	100	4	0	95	11	1	6	300	8	10	0	45	6	30	50
Soy Yogurt (227 g)	1 cntnr	150	4	0	30	22	1	6	0	12	0	50	30	0	30	0
Veggie pattie - Chik	1 Pattie	140	5	0	590	16	2	8	280	1	0	0	2	10	0	20
Veggie pattie - Griller	1 Pattie	130	6	0	260	5	2	15	130	0	0	0	4	10	0	45
Veggie pattie - Turk'y	1 Pattie	90	5	0	390	7	5	9	270	0	0	0	4	15	0	0
Vegs - sweet potato raw 5 oz	1 Med	100	0	0	70	23	4	2	440	7	120	30	4	4	0	0

DNS 15—Vegan Labels

Total Daily Nutrition	Serving	1480	31	49	2410	217	19	41	1507	122	115	57	50	43	40	$0.00
Based on 1500 Calories	Size or	Calories	50gm	<300mg	<2400mg	225gm	20mg	38gm	2625mg	Sugar	5000IU	60mg	1000mg	18mg	400IU	Average
Cholesterol & Sodium	Amount	Total	Total Fat	Choles- terol	Sodium	Carbs	Fiber	Protein	Potas- sium	grams	Vit A	Vit C	Calcium	Iron	Vit D	Cost Per Serving
same all calorie levels											Percent totals at the top of these columns are for the 100% on the NF label needed at 2,000 calories					
Breakfast																
Sugar in coffee	3 tps	45	0	0	0	4	0	0	0	4	0	0	0	0	0	
Creamer in coffee	4 tps	60	3	0	15	9	0	0	0	7	0	0	0	0	0	
Tropical fruit	1/2 C	60	0	0	5	15	1	0	160	14	10	45	0	0	0	
Oatmeal, walnut,raisin,dates	1 pkt	140	3	0	190	27	3	3	140	11	20	0	10	20	0	
Walnuts in oatmeal	1/8 C	190	2	0	0	4	2	4	125	0	0	0	2	4	0	
Raisins in oatmeal	1/4 C	130	0	0	10	31	2	1	310	29	0	0	2	6	0	
Lunch																
Soup, chicken & vegetable	1 C	110	2	15	710	17	3	6	0	3	25	2	0	4	0	
Crackers	4 pieces	70	3	0	125	9	0	0	0	1	0	0	0	0	0	
Applesauce, chunky	1/2 C	90	0	0	10	23	2	0	0	19	0	0	0	0	0	
Dinner																
Tuna, Albacore	1/4 C	70	2	25	190	0	0	13	130	0	0	0	0	0	15	
Mayonnaise, light	1 Tbsp	35	4	4	125	0	0	3	0	0	0	0	0	0	0	
Bread, whole wheat	2 slices	120	2	0	220	24	4	3	0	1	0	0	2	4	0	
Salt, 45% iodine	1/8 tsp	0	0	0	295	0	0	0	0	0	0	0	0	0	0	
Vegetables, mixed	1/2 C	45	0	0	260	10	2	2	200	3	50	0	2	2	0	
Milk, skim	1 C	90	0	5	135	13	0	9	420	12	10	10	30	0	25	
Snack																
Cookies	3	225	10	0	120	31	0	0	22	18	0	0	0	3	0	

DNS 16—Judy's Food Day

Total Daily Nutrition		1502	58	107	2505	240	20	69	3835	136	167	200	192	39	110	$5.11
Based on 1500 Calories	Serving	Calories	50gm	<300mg	<2400mg	225gm	20mg	38gm	2625mg	Sugar	5000IU	60mg	1000mg	18mg	400IU	Average
Cholesterol & Sodium	Size or	Total	Total	Choles-	Sodium	Carbs	Fiber	Protein	Potas-	grams	Vit A	Vit C	Calcium	Iron	Vit D	Cost Per
same all calorie levels	Amount		Fat	terol					sium		Percent totals at the top of these columns are for the 100% on the NF label needed at 2,000 calories						Serving
Breakfast																
Orange Juice, 100% fresh squeezed	1 C	110	0	0	0	26	0	2	450	22	0	120	35	0	25	$0.47
Banana	1 Med	105	26	3	0	26	3	2	422	14	2	10	0	1	0	$0.21
Cereal, Oats, Raisin, Dates, Walnuts	1 pkt	140	3	0	190	27	3	3	140	11	20	0	10	20	0	$0.24
Milk, fat-free	1 Cup	90	0	5	135	13	0	9	420	12	10	10	30	0	25	$0.23
Lunch																
Chicken, canned in water	1/4 C	60	1	30	200	0	0	13	0	0	0	0	0	2	0	$0.51
Bread, 100% whole wheat	1 Slice	60	1	0	110	12	2	3	0	2	0	0	4	4	0	$0.12
Salad Dressing, mayonnaise light	1 Tbsp	35	4	4	125	0	0	0	0	0	0	0	0	0	0	$0.07
Cheese, American Singles	1 Slice	70	5	15	220	2	0	4	0	1	4	0	25	0	10	$0.11
Potato, canned sliced potatoes	2/3 C	70	0	0	280	14	2	1	290	0	0	20	4	2	0	$0.46
Canned, carrots, green beans, peas, corn, lima beans	1/2 C	50	0	0	310	10	3	2	190	3	60	6	2	4	0	$0.25
Milk, fat-free	1 Cup	90	0	5	135	13	0	9	420	12	10	10	30	0	25	$0.23
Dinner																
Soup, chicken & vegetables	1 Cup	90	1	10	410	16	3	5	920	4	30	4	4	4	0	$0.95
Crackers, Club crackers	4 crkrs	70	3	0	125	9	0	1	0	1	0	0	0	0	0	$0.12
Apple, raw 2 3/4 " with skin	1 Med	72	0	0	0	19	4	4	148	14	15	10	8	0	0	$0.33
Milk, fat-free	1 Cup	90	0	5	135	13	0	9	420	12	10	10	30	0	25	$0.23
Snack																
Cookies, golden double stuf	2 Cks	150	7	0	80	21	0	0	15	12	0	0	0	2	0	$0.19
Ice Cream, cherry vanilla	1/2 C	150	7	30	50	19	0	3	0	16	6	0	10	0	0	$0.39

DNS 17—$5 Average Food Cost at 1,500 Calorie Level

Total Daily Nutrition Based on 2000 Calories Cholesterol & Sodium same all calorie levels.	Serving Size or Amount	Calories Total 2042	Total Fat 70 / 65 gm	Choles-terol 0 / <300mg	Sodium 2635 / <2400mg	Carbs 258 / 300gm	Fiber 54 / 25 mg	Protein 78 / 50gm	Potas-sium 3233 / 3500mg	Sugar grams 127	Vit A 171 / 5000IU	Vit C 182 / 60mg	Calcium 165 / 1000mg	Iron 102 / 18mg	Vit D 85 / 400IU	Vit B12 170 / 6mcg
											Percent totals at the top of these columns are for the 100% on the NF label needed at 2,000					
Cereal, Raisin Bran	1 C	190	1	0	210	46	7	5	390	18	10	0	2	25	0	25
Soy Milk	1 C	100	4	0	95	11	1	6	300	8	10	0	45	6	30	50
Fruit - Apple, raw 2 3/4 " with skin	1 Med	72	0	0	0	19	4	4	148	14	15	10	8	0	0	0
Cheese - vegan	1 Oz	90	7	0	260	7	1	1	0	0	0	0	0	0	0	0
Veggie pattie - Griller	1 Pattie	130	6	0	260	5	2	15	130	0	0	0	4	10	0	45
Vegs - sweet peas - canned	1/2 C	70	5	0	370	12	3	4	105	6	6	20	2	8	0	0
Bread - 100% whole wheat	1 Slice	60	1	0	110	12	2	3	0	2	0	0	4	4	0	0
Peanut Butter, natural super chunk	2 Tbsp	190	17	0	125	6	2	7	0	3	0	0	0	4	0	0
Veggie pattie - Turky	1 Pattie	90	5	0	390	7	5	9	270	0	0	0	4	15	0	0
Fruit - Juice, 100% squeezed from fresh oranges with calcium & vitamin D	1 C	110	0	0	0	26	0	2	450	22	0	120	35	0	25	0
Vegs - sweet potato raw 5 oz	1 Med	100	0	0	70	23	4	2	440	7	120	30	4	4	0	0
Beans - baked	1/2 C	150	1	0	530	30	8	6	390	8	0	2	6	10	0	0
Bread - 100% whole wheat	1 Slice	60	1	0	110	12	2	3	0	2	0	0	4	4	0	0
Soy Milk	1 C	100	4	0	95	11	1	6	300	8	10	0	45	6	30	50
Fruit - Raisins, regular & golden raisins	1/4 C	130	0	0	10	31	2	1	310	29	0	0	2	6	0	0
Soy Ice Cream	1 C	400	18	0	0	0	10	4	0	0	0	0	0	0	0	0

DNS 18—Vegan's Food Day

REFERENCES

U.S. Department of Health and Human Services and U.S. Department of Agriculture. *Dietary Guidelines for Americans, 2005.* 6th Edition, Washington, DC: U.S. Government Printing Office, January 2005

U.S. Department of Agriculture and U.S. Department of Health and Human Services. *Dietary Guidelines for Americans, 2010.* 7th Edition, Washington, DC: U.S. Government Printing Office, December 2010

About the Author

Judy Webb Brewster has been writing since 1986. She has received awards for her fiction, non-fiction, and poetry. Her work has appeared in The Kansas City Star, the Pitch Magazine, and movie reviews in The Sun Newspaper. She enjoys sharing her unique view of life with her readers.

She held a full-time job while acquiring a BBA in Business Administration, and in her spare time she was on stage, and back stage, at the local community theatres. She has held positions on several boards including President of the HOA board where she lived. She spent a few years in her brother's country western band playing three keyboards.

Today her extra time is spent enjoying her family, friends, golfing, bicycling, and taking ballroom dance lessons.

www.closeenoughnutrition.com